MEAT IS FOR PUSSIES

———

A How-To Guide for Dudes Who
Want to Get Fit, Kick Ass, and Take Names

Meat Is for Pussies

John Joseph

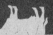

HARPER WAVE

HarperCollins books may be purchased for educational, business, or sales promotional use. For information, please e-mail the Special Markets Department at SPsales@harpercollins.com.

Originally self-published, in a different form, as *Meat is for Pussies* in the United States in 2010 by Crush Books.

FIRST EDITION

Designed by *John Kapenga, Michael Yamagata, and William Ruoto*

Library of Congress Cataloging-in-Publication Data

Joseph, John (punk rock musician)

Meat is for pussies : a how-to guide for dudes who want to get fit, kick ass, and take names / John Joseph.

      pages cm

ISBN 978-0-06-232032-2 (hardback)

1. Veganism. 2. Vegetarianism. 3. Men—Nutrition. 4. Men—Health and hygiene. 5. Physical fitness for men. I. Title.

RM236.J67   2014

613.2'622—dc23   2014013846

14 15 16 17 18   OV/RRD   10 9 8 7 6 5 4 3 2

This book is dedicated to all of the warriors for truth,
freedom, and health worldwide.

CONTENTS

FOREWORD BY RICH ROLL   X

INTRODUCTION   **XIX**

CHAPTER 1
GET SCARED STRAIGHT   1

CHAPTER 2
DUDE, THE PARTY'S OVER   13

CHAPTER 3
THE GREAT FOOD BAMBOOZLE   27

CHAPTER 4
DON'T BE THEIR HUMAN LAB RATS   39

CONTENTS

CHAPTER 5
THE REAL WMDs   49

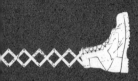

CHAPTER 6
KICK CANCER (AND OTHER DISEASES)   59
IN THE NUTS

CHAPTER 7
GET THE POISON OUT   71

LIVING PROOF   83

CHAPTER 8
THE BULLSHIT PROTEIN MYTH   93

CHAPTER 9
DIETS ARE FOR JERK-OFFS   107

CHAPTER 10
FREE YOUR MIND, BODY,   **125**
AND YOUR ASS
WILL FOLLOW

CHAPTER 11
TRANSITION TO HEALTH IN   **137**
FOUR EASY STEPS

CHAPTER 12
30 DAYS TO ROCK SOLID   **149**

CHAPTER 13
SUPER BADASS RECIPES   **181**

AFTERWORD BY FRED BISCI   **249**
ACKNOWLEDGMENTS   **253**
APPENDIX   **257**
NOTES   **278**
INDEX   **284**

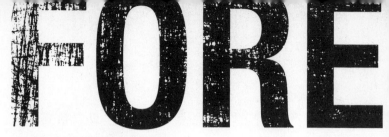

BY RICH ROLL

You may think that *Meat Is for Pussies* is a book about why we should remove animal products from our diet. Certainly it is that. But between the lines, I see so much more.

From a survivor who has gone to hell and back, this book is a manifesto on the ethos of masculinity—what it truly means to be a man of strength and purpose in modern society. A finely tuned primer on course-correcting our upside-down cultural priorities. A road map for living a legacy-worthy life of meaning. And a call to action to once and for all seize control of our health and our lives so we can unlock and unleash the best part of who we are and what we leave behind in this short, precious life.

We live in a curious time when literally *everything* has become about facilitating comfort and ease. Our cultural mandate has become the elimination of obstacles and challenges, the brass-ring achievement defined by leisure—a life free of stress, pain, hardship, and struggle. Meanwhile, our focus is keenly placed on the accumulation of *stuff*, most of which is specifically designed to make our lives easier, more comfortable. We are brainwashed into believing that flat-screen TVs, high-speed Internet, car seat warmers, 401(k)s, fast food, and designer pharmaceuticals

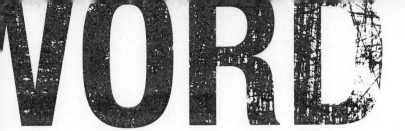

for every conceivable ailment, imagined or otherwise, hold the key to our identity and ultimately our happiness.

The United States is the most prosperous nation in the world, and yet our *citizenship* has been comprehensively reduced to *consumerism*. A culture in which our primary directive is the quest to accumulate this *stuff*, or at least more than our friends and neighbors. *Buy and ye shall be happy.*

But what have we truly purchased? In the words of my favorite writer, Henry David Thoreau, "The mass of men lead lives of quiet desperation." Our lives prostrate at the altar of the false gods of our instant-gratification society. A culture of emasculated drones more depressed, obese, diseased, stressed, lethargic, medicated, generally unhappy, and overall unfulfilled than any other culture on the planet. An entrenched, self-perpetuating cycle then ensues that drives us to further escape, salving our pain and disillusionment with unhealthy food choices, television, video games, alcohol, illicit drugs and pharmaceuticals, shopping, gambling, or unhappy relationships; you name it. The hole never gets filled, of course—it just grows deeper. More hungry. A bottomless pit into which we willingly jump. A succumbing, in the ethos of Thoreau, to the *delusion of need*. A profound lunacy that is bankrupting our souls and decimating our planet.

Most of all, we're *sick*. Sicker than we've ever been, on both an individual and a planetary level. And if we continue along this path, the prognosis is bleak.

In truth, we're in the midst of an almost unspeakable, unsustainable health-care and environmental crisis. Despite our spending more than $22 billion a year on fad diet and weight loss products, 70 percent of all Americans are obese or overweight. Childhood obesity rates are through the roof. One out of every three deaths in America is attributable to heart disease, our number-one killer. And by 2030, 30 percent of Americans will be diabetic or pre-diabetic. In response, we have become indentured servants to the pharmaceutical industry, popping pills that effectively mask symptoms but more often than not do little or nothing to prevent or cure our underlying chronic ailments. Meanwhile, our factory farm system is irrevocably depleting our soil. And livestock harvesting is polluting our bodies with saturated fat, hormones, pesticides, and genetically modified organisms (GMOs), all while destroying the environment at an unfathomable rate.

Our reaction? Grab a beer, pop a pill, order a pizza, and leave me alone on the Barcalounger because *Duck Dynasty* is on the TiVo. No wonder we're so screwed.

True happiness is an inside job unlocked only by cracking through the protective crust of our social armor to delve deeply and honestly into what drives us. Happiness is forged through struggles, challenges, and failures to elucidate personal growth, self-knowledge, and ultimately fulfillment. It is achieved through selfless service to others, as well as to the authentic self within. This is hardly a new concept, and yet it is one that eludes most people. Intellectually we understand this to be the case but most of us simply shirk away, slinking back into our chimerical zone of comfort and denial like an addict to the opium den. A world of conforming to societal expectations, doing what we're told. Buying stuff and keeping quiet. Indeed, *The Matrix*.

I know this because I've been there—I had to discover all of this the hard way. I have decades under my belt of medicating myself in every conceivable way. Drugs, alcohol, fast food, you name it—I was a black belt at "checking out"—a path that took me to some very dark and desperate places. In 2006, I was a classic couch potato. Fifty pounds overweight, overworked, lethargic, depressed, and subsisting almost entirely on what I like to call the *window diet*—if it could be handed to me through my car window at the drive-through, I ate it.

Then paid for it.

The good news is that there is a solution. A solution that begins and ends with what you put in your mouth. John Joseph gets it. And this, people, is what *Meat Is for Pussies* is really all about.

When I adopted a plant-based diet at the age of forty, it was out of sheer pain, utter desperation, and acute fear of the heart attack that almost certainly loomed in my not too distant future. At the time, my goals were modest. All I wanted was to live. Lose a little weight. Feel better. And be able to enjoy my children at their energy level. Personally, I didn't think it would work. And I'm the last guy on earth who ever thought he would call himself that dreaded five-letter word: *vegan*.

Astoundingly, this simple change led me to a path I never could have predicted in a million years. A journey of not just athletic prowess but self-discovery that has given my life true meaning and purpose. A journey that has taught me how to be a man. A real man.

Not only did this shift in dietary preference repair my health; it provided vitality beyond anything I could imagine. I found myself so energized, I resumed a modest fitness protocol just to burn off all the extra energy. In short order, my weight dropped from 210 to 162, what I weighed in high school. Amazed, I began to look for an athletic challenge, fueled by a singular question: *If I could suddenly feel so good after decades of abusing my body with drugs, alcohol, and fast food, just how resilient is the human body?*

People would constantly tell me that I could never be an athlete without consuming animal protein. My body told me differently. And just two years later I found myself neck and neck with some of the best endurance athletes in the world.

Despite never previously having raced a bike or been a competitive runner, in 2009 I finished sixth at the Ultraman World Championships—a three-day, 320-mile, double-Ironman distance triathlon that circumnavigates the entire Big Island of Hawaii—widely considered one of the most daunting endurance challenges on the planet. The following year I continued to defy middle age and push the boundaries of human capability by becoming the first person (along with fellow vegan athlete Jason Lester) to complete EPIC5: an über-endurance adventure in which I finished five Ironman-distance triathlons on five Hawaiian islands in less than a week. I was forty-four years old.

My question had been answered. *The human body is far more resilient than you can possibly imagine, capable of truly astounding things when treated properly.*

These accomplishments landed me on CNN and the pages of magazines like *Men's Fitness*, which awarded me the title of one of the "25 Fittest Men in the World," eventually culminating in a book deal for my memoir, *Finding Ultra*, and a life now devoted to wellness advocacy.

I do not detail these accomplishments to pad my ego and I definitely don't stand on a pedestal. I stumble often, and almost every step in my personal evolution has been forged entirely out of the crucible of pain. Instead, I relate these facts of my experience solely to highlight the remarkable extent to which my life transformed in every conceivably way since removing animal products from my diet.

Not everyone wants to be an ultra-endurance athlete. I get that. The point is that we all have a better, healthier, more authentic version of ourselves locked within, yearning to be expressed. If I could change so drastically, I know for a fact this powerful reality resides within all of us.

Plant-based nutrition didn't just repair my health. It was the key that unlocked my heart. It was the catalyst that made my entire crazy journey possible by unleashing an internal personal power I never thought possible to actualize the best, most authentic version of myself. To echo Thoreau, *we need not lead lives of quiet desperation*. You can break the chains of enslavement to take control of your health, fitness, and destiny. And no matter what your circumstances, it's never too late.

Heart disease, diabetes, obesity, and cancer are playing for keeps. But there is a solution. In fact, 90 percent of Western disease is preventable or reversible through simple diet and lifestyle alteration. Plant-based nutrition is the true path to sustainable long-term wellness for both the individual and the planet at large.

It's not a fad. The plant power revolution is here, people. It's for real. And it's available to you. You only have to do one thing—decide.

I'll leave you with this. Set aside your preconceived notions, take John's hand, and make the leap. Challenge yourself and your assumptions. Let go of habits that don't serve you. Embrace the struggle. In fact, welcome it with every fiber of your being. Throw yourself into the muck, put yourself on the line, and stare it right in the face. But most of all? Dream big.

Whatever the result, seize the opportunity to learn something about yourself. Apply it. *Grow*. Then watch everything about your life change.

Or as John would say, *don't be a pussy*.

Peace + Plants,
Rich Roll

NTRO

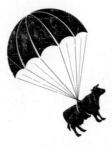

INTRODUCTION

Who propagated this bullshit that meat makes you macho? My guess is it's the same big business assholes who told you the Marlboro Man was a stud. Well, eating defenseless animals doesn't make you tough, numb-nuts, it makes you a coward. You wanna eat meat? Then instead of purchasing factory-killed, slickly packaged animal parts, have some balls and tear one down with your bare hands and rip it apart. I guarantee you'll find out how much of a pussy you are when you get your ass handed to you like some idiot on *When Animals Attack*. I've met so many weight-lifter Neanderthals over the years that were like, "Yo, men need meat, it makes us strong and aggressive." Or my favorite, the protein myth: "If you don't eat meat, you don't get enough protein." As if dead, rotting carcasses were the only sources of protein. In reality, there are dozens of sources that don't require systematic incarceration, torture, and slaughter. And as far as aggression, I know some vegetarians who will rip your fuckin' head off in a New York minute.

I'm sick of these people who are ignorant of the facts—the kind that diss vegetarians because we care about animals or the environment. These fools have bought into the lies and propaganda put out there by the douche bags running the meat industry—the same douche bags who happen to be some of the country's most powerful lobbyists. There was that bullshit ad campaign that they ran a while ago: "Beef, it's what's for dinner." Yeah, beef's for dinner, but colon cancer, arterial sclerosis, high blood pressure, animal cruelty, and a destroyed planet are your karmic dessert.

Now, just so we get off on the right foot, I want to fill you in on my background. I'm not some new-age health nut who's trying to get you to eat your sprouts. Most of those people make me want to puke. To be honest with you, I don't blame you carnivorous fuckers for looking at the majority of vegetarians and wanting nothing to do with a meat-free diet. The truth is that I've had a harder life than most. I've survived orphanages, abusive foster homes, the mean streets of New York City in the mid-1970s, shootings, stabbings, lockups, drug addiction, homelessness, the music business . . . the list goes on (you can read all about it in my autobiography, *The Evolution of a Cro-Magnon*). Anyway, if anyone knows a thing or two about being tough and fighting on, it's me. So prepare your brain cells for a no-holds-barred, New York–style beat-down on real health and real nutrition. Trust me, I'm not pulling any punches.

The first thing meat-eaters say to me is, "Damn, you're a vegetarian?" I know what they mean. Some of the vegetarians I see look like sickly, weak-as-fuck string beans. Why? Because they eat shitty overprocessed foods, avoid working out, and drink and smoke to excess. But I've been at this for thirty-three years, and I'm as physical as they come. On any given day I run ten miles, hit the gym, pump some weights, take a fifty-mile bike ride and a long swim. As a matter of fact, I just finished two full Ironman triathlons and an Olympic distance in the last year, and when I ran the Marine Corps Marathon in 2007 I beat every fucker in my group, some of whom weren't even half my age. When they crossed the finish line and found me cooled down and enjoying a snack, all they could say was, "Damn, old man." Now at fifty-one, I'm still a stage-diving, triathlon-loving maniac, and I attribute this endurance to two things: consistency in training and, most important, proper food choices. Over the years I've worked out at a lot of gyms and watched a lot of trainers instructing people, and most of those idiots don't know shit about nutrition. I mean, at one old-school gym on the Lower East Side a bodybuilder told me that Alpo burgers are a great source of protein. He said that if it's good enough for his pit bull, it's good enough for him. That's an extreme case, but you get my point. If you aren't hip to what the fuck you're putting in your body, it's like trying to light a fire in the pouring rain.

The first thing I'm gonna do is explain what all that shit you're ingesting is doing to your body. Then I'll present you with healthy alternatives, show you how to take control of your health, even give you kick-ass recipes from some amazing chef friends of mine, and provide a thirty-day workout plan created just for you by Aaron Drogoszewski, who trains professional athletes as well as yours truly. Notice I don't use the word *diet*; diets are for pussies. If you're tired of being on one of those Atkins, Jenny Craig, or Weight Watchers pussy diets, man up and read on. On the other hand, if you're happy with calorie counting like a fat chick in her Curves class, return my book and continue on with your chronic pussyism.

I decided to pen this book because all the people I've advised over the years keep saying the same thing after they made the switch to a plant-based diet: "Damn, bro, this is easier than I thought." No shit, guys, this ain't rocket science. I've spent more than half my life learning about plant-based eating and experiencing the benefits firsthand. So I know my stuff when it comes to optimum health, nutrition, and training a lot better than some of the so-called experts. And as far as doctors are concerned, it seems like most of them don't talk much about prevention. Nah, they'd rather write you a prescription for the drug companies' very expensive medicine to treat the symptoms. There's no money in the cure. And there's a whole lot less funding for research on disease prevention using whole foods as medicine than there is money being poured into the pharmaceutical industry.

According to Gladys Block, PhD, a recent epidemiological study has shown much lower cancer rates in people whose diets are rich in fruits and vegetables.[1] Guess what? The meat industry doesn't want you to know that. Shit, lots of people would lose their jobs if you were eating healthy. That's why Texas cattlemen sued Oprah back in 1996 when she had Howard Lyman, a brilliant vegetarian activist who wrote the great book *The Mad Cowboy*, on her show.[2] When he told her that the United States was in danger of an outbreak of mad cow disease, she said she'd never eat another hamburger. Then, as they say, the excrement hit the fan.

The key to learning is to keep an open mind and try new things, so I'll show you what has worked best for me and those I've passed this info on to over the years. Make no mistake about it: my intention is to get you to stop eating meat for your own sake. It's easier than you think, especially since meat-free foods, prepared properly, taste amazing. The easy-to-make, nutrient-rich meals and super-food recommendations in the back of this book will jump-start your metabolism and kick your libido into overdrive. Ah, now I've got your attention, don't I? Read on and you'll learn about even more benefits.

With my approach, I always try to be a little philo-sophical. To quote Eleanor Roosevelt, "Somewhere along the line of development we discover what we really are, and then we make our real decision for which we are responsi-ble. Make that decision primarily for yourself because you can never really live anyone else's life, not even your own child's. The influence you exert is through your own life and what you become yourself."

Exactly, fellas, it's all about dedication and making lifelong changes. If you begin to make better food choices and combine it with a solid exercise regimen, you'll become a force to be reckoned with. If you breeze through this book and ignore everything I have to say, you'll continue on your path toward debilitating illness, devastating weak-ness, and inevitable pussyism. The choice is yours. Every journey starts with a first step, and the first step of this journey is to understand how the harmful effects of eating meat and living a sedentary lifestyle will turn you into a PUSSY dependent upon the pharmaceutical companies' drugs to keep you alive. If that's your thing, read no further; this book isn't for you. But if you're like most people I talk to across the globe who are sick and tired of being sick and tired, read on because I can guarantee you with 100 percent certainty that if you apply what's in the pages of this book to your life, it will be a game changer.

GET

SCARED
STRAIGHT

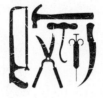

CHAPTER 1

GET SCARED STRAIGHT

Growing up in the 1970s, I was a kid who hustled on the streets. Eventually, the long arm of the law caught up with me and sent me upstate to a juvenile detention center. The brass there took me to Rahway State Prison in New Jersey, for Scared Straight, a new program designed to scare the living shit out of kids and force changes in their lives. They had these lifers—guys doing time for murder, rape, and a slew of other horrific crimes—who would tell you what it's like to be incarcerated in places like Rahway or New York's Fishkill maximum-security prison and watch your life waste away. Let me tell you something: it worked. I changed my tune after meeting those scary fuckers. So now I'm going to conduct my own session of Scared Straight. Lucky for you, I'm not going to scream at you, make you give me your sneakers, slap you upside the head, or spit in your face. What I am going to do is explain what's coming tomorrow if you don't make some crucial changes in your dietary practices today. The dude with one eye who wanted to make me his bitch got to me, and what you're about to read is gonna get to you.

DIGEST THIS

———

Let's take a look at some of the leading PREVENT-ABLE causes of death in the United States every year. In 2010 cancer and heart disease claimed almost 600,000 lives apiece, stroke almost 130,000, and diabetes almost 70,000.[3] And these numbers just scratch the surface of how sick we really are as a society. Disease is running rampant, wreaking havoc on our lives and the lives of our loved ones.

Just stop and think for a moment about all those people, almost 1.4 million of us, who could have gone on to live longer, healthier lives. Guess what? You have the power to protect yourself and your health, if you change the course you're on right now.

Do you think the drug companies want you to get better? Hell no. They want you to stay a sick, whining mama's boy so you can fuel an industry whose global sales are more than $300 billion a year, and expected to balloon up to $400 billion within three years.[4] You don't see drug dealers telling their customers, "Yo, man, I think you need to go to rehab." Not gonna happen, Slick. We're addicts, and sooner or later we're going to crash. How bad is it, you ask? Let me put it to you like this: never before in the history of planet earth has the food we're eating, the products we are using, and the lifestyles we're leading had a bigger impact on our health. Simply put, we're killing ourselves.

We're in so deep, we can't even see straight. Here's an example of how blind we've become. Recently a KFC franchise advertised a promotion to help fight juvenile diabetes. If you bought a half gallon of soda, what they call the "Mega Jug," which contains a whopping 800 calories and 56 spoonfuls of white sugar, they would donate one whole fucking dollar to the Juvenile Diabetes Research Foundation.[5] In other words, help find a cure for type 1 diabetes by putting yourself at greater risk of contracting type 2 diabetes. Who comes up with this shit?

It's no wonder the United States spends two and a half times what the average country spends on health-care costs. That's a whopping $8,233 per person.[6] Here's the thing, though: many of these medical problems could go away if we just changed our dietary and lifestyle habits. Health is the key to a long and enjoyable life, and as you read on you'll see the need for us to stop being pussies—and that eliminating meat and eating real foods from plants is the way to do that.

Let's start with the basics. You ready? Put on your thinking cap and answer this: Why is it that we know more about health than ever before, but so many of us are fat, sick, and unhealthy? Let me tell you why. First off, we're subjecting ourselves (and the earth) to the largest toxic load in the history of the planet. We're organic, just like the planet; so when we poison the planet's water, air, and soil, we're poisoning ourselves. When you support the meat industry by purchasing the products of its chemically treated, drugged-up, and genetically engineered ranching and farming (nicely sealed for you in shiny, nonbiodegradable packaging), you're fucking yourself up. And guess what? You're also fucking up the entire planet.

Second, we're willingly ingesting foodstuffs that are pure poison to the body. These foods are overprocessed, overcooked, bursting with saturated fat, and loaded with chemicals and preservatives. In fact, most of what we eat is devoid of any nutritional value whatsoever. We simply eat empty calories so our fat fucking guts feel full. Now throw in cigarettes, alcohol, prescription medications, and the stress of everyday life and you've got a recipe for disaster. Do you guys remember "the Juiceman," Jay Kordich, from those infomercials in the eighties? He used to do an amazing experiment. He'd have an audience member come up and put everything he ingested over the course of the day into a clear bowl. First in went the greasy bacon, fried eggs, white toast, coffee, and cigarettes consumed at breakfast. Next came lunch, which consisted of french fries, a hamburger, soda, and more cigarettes. Dinner was Kentucky Fried Chicken, a big piece of cake, coffee, a few drinks, and what else but an after-dinner stogie. Jay's point was this: that bowl represented our stomachs, and when he held that shit up and swirled it around, it became a deadly toxic soup. We do that to our bodies every single day, day in and day out, and still our bodies go on functioning and fighting. But one day soon—and believe me, it's coming—all of that poison will catch up with you and you'll join the rank and file of people suffering from those killer diseases. One day, meat and processed foods will turn you into a feeble pussy.

GET YOUR SHIT TOGETHER

Now you may say, "Man, it's too much of an inconvenience to do all that." Well, talk to my friend who had to go on kidney dialysis three days a week for five hours each day because a combination of taking a bunch of prescription medications and a lifetime of eating bad foods ravaged his kidneys. Or visit a cancer ward where people are having their colons or cancerous polyps ripped out of their assholes. Or go to a drugstore and watch the faces of the people coming to pick up their three hundred dollars' worth of medicine every week. Health is an investment, and staying healthy becomes far easier once you get serious.

So how do we get off this train? It's simple: start gradually. Substitute that toxic breakfast for some fruit, oatmeal, and whole grain toast. For lunch, get a veggie burger, some salad, and a raw green juice. Buy some cookbooks that give you options for plant-based meals (check out the Appendix on page 257 for my recommendations) or go out for dinner to a veggie-friendly restaurant. Little by little, replace processed foods with organic, whole foods. Drink as much fresh-pressed fruit juice, green juice, and filtered water as you can. And stay away from any and all animal proteins.

I'm going to tell you something you probably already know deep down inside: you're eating like a lazy fuckin' pussy. That has to change, and it will. Want to know why? You've already taken the first step by reading this book. The first step in drug rehab is admitting that you're an addict. And even though I'm busting your chops like those guys at Rahway State Prison, it's only because I care about you the same way they cared about me. I'm gonna teach you about little changes that lead to incredible results, but you've gotta remember that longevity is the key. Don't be like one of those fuckers who latches on to a fad diet, only to burn out shortly after. What I'm talking about is a life-long change, so I don't mince words: stop making excuses and get off your fat ass.

It's all about teamwork, so you should surround yourself with people who aren't addicted to bad food. Just like how Narcotics Anonymous tells you to steer clear of people, places, and things that remind you of drugs, I'm telling you to avoid those junk food junkies. You should be afraid. In fact, be very afraid. If you're eating breakfast, lunch, or dinner with junk food junkies, you're going right back to square one.

And be warned . . . anytime you break away from the status quo and try and live outside the box, you will have people telling you what you're doing is crazy. Oh yes, there will be many who will want to do battle with you, who have little or no understanding of nutrition, but yet feel qualified to tell you it's a big mistake to go plant based. They'll call you on their cell phones and say they heard this and that, all while standing in line at the drugstore to fill their bottles of medication that they need because they're eating such wonderful diets. So here's the thing you can take comfort in: what's in this book not only has been tested by me as a living lab rat, but is also the product of reviewing all of the latest clinical research on diet and nutrition. There are no snake oil salesmen here. The doctors and experts I've interviewed all have degrees; what they don't have is a hidden agenda or an interest in keeping you sick for profit. Their business is to heal you and get you off those dangerous medications once and for all.

Do not, I repeat, *do not* be afraid of failure. If you're afraid, you'll never even start your journey. Don't be a sucker who stands around the water cooler and lies through his teeth like, "Yeah, Bob, one day I'm gonna run that damn marathon or take a shot at a triathlon," but that day never comes. Even worse are the procrastinators who make themselves feel better by thinking, "Yeah, I'll run it. I'm going to get in that first jog one day . . . I've just got so much crap to do today. I'll start tomorrow." These chumps may even buy new sneakers, lay out a nice jogging suit the night before, and set their alarm clock for an early run. But when that clock goes off the next morning they send it flying off the night table, roll over, fart, scratch their balls, curse the day, and lie there letting their mind beat them down. Pussies swear by this routine because their fear of failure is kicking the living shit out of them. It even invites resistance, its best friend, to come over and get a few kicks in.

When I started writing books and screenplays, the first thing I learned is this: never, ever let resistance beat you.

Resistance is a son of a bitch. As Steven Pressfield writes in *The War of Art*: "Resistance has no conscience. It will pledge anything to get a deal then double-cross you as soon as your back is turned. If you take resistance at its word, you deserve everything you get. Resistance is always lying and always full of shit." I like to think of resistance as my worst enemy. Is my worst enemy ever gonna tell me to do something that's beneficial for me? Hell no. You've gotta be willing to fail to a degree. It's part of the learning experience.

Hemingway said that the first draft of anything is complete shit, so don't expect perfection right out of the box. That's not being realistic; it's actually resistance looking to con you, break you, and make you feel inadequate. Ask any fit person how long it took them to get their body to where it is today and I'm sure they'll tell you it took years. If you don't put your ego aside, the path will be very difficult. I slipped up in the beginning, but I didn't quit. Slipping up and quitting are two entirely different concepts. If you're determined to get better and improve your health, you will. We've dealt with bad habits most of our lives, and they don't go away or stop tempting us overnight. Everything in this world is based on desire. We're talking about the desire to make changes and the desire to take risks. Is this desire to create a new and healthy life a risk? Hell fuckin' yes it is. That's why all the regular, meat-eating pussies would rather continue leading their bodies on this warpath. They're scared to face who they really are and would rather have a few cold ones with resistance, their old drinking buddy.

But anything of value is proportional to the risk you take to achieve it—the greater the value, the greater the risk. You may lose hangout time with some of your friends at first—big deal. But as they start seeing how great you look and feel, they'll want to know how you got there. And when you have real friendships that grow from positive vibes, you can work together to get healthy.

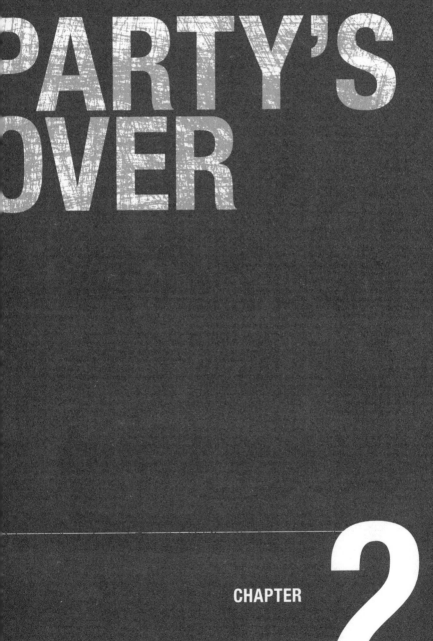

DUDE, THE

PARTY'S
OVER

CHAPTER **2**

DUDE, THE PARTY'S OVER

Health Is the New Black

Look, I'm not going to preach to you about how you like to have a good time, because that's not my thing. I judge no one. What you do for fun is your own business—well, that is, unless you bring your drunken asshole antics into my personal space. Then we got issues. But anyway, since you are trying to better yourself, before we go any further we need to address a few things. Point blank, if you want a fighting chance at achieving your ultimate level of health and fitness, you have to take a step back and look at the daily choices you're making.

Now, from my own personal experience of living in New York City and traveling around the globe for the last thirty-plus years I've learned a few things about the party-ing lifestyle. I've also lost a shitload of friends and family members, which was quite sobering. And as a matter of fact, that's exactly what I'm getting at . . . sobriety. Again, not judging—I've been there, too. I was a crackhead in the late eighties. You could say I know the drill.

While I was using drugs I was a bit of an anomaly be-cause I was also trying to be a super-healthy dude. As I was quoted saying in *Triathlete* magazine, "I'd smoke crack all night and still go get wheatgrass juice in the morning." Hon-estly, that's probably why I didn't die with the amount of poison I was ingesting. I'd smoke crack and be up for days, then I'd have to pop pills to come down off the high and be able to sleep. By day I was like, "The enzymes contained in organic raw foods balance your pH level and help to pre-vent cancer by reducing acidity in the body." Then at night it was, "Yo, kid, lemme get twenty bucks, they got them jumbo fucking vials of crack up the block." That's no joke.

The sad truth is addiction runs in my family. My pops was an alcoholic and my brother suffered the same fate as well, being a pill head and alcoholic for the last twenty-plus years. Matter of fact, we almost lost him to heart disease as his bad habits finally caught up to him. They always do. Let me tell you, when you are face-to-face with an impend-ing early death, it's definitely a sobering wake-up call.

So why am I airing my dirty laundry here? First, because

if it helps one person avoid what I went through, it's worth it, and, second, because I want you to know I'm not telling you this shit from a pulpit but rather down in the trenches with you. I wake up and I meditate every day to maintain my sobriety. I know that one hit, one drink, or one pill and I'm right back where I was and that place was complete and total hell. Honestly, I shouldn't even be alive with all the insane shit I did when I was using. Robbing armed coke dealers. Being in a drug house that was riddled with gunfire because someone I was freebasing with stole a pound of coke from the cocaine cowboy Cuban dealers in Miami. High-speed chases with cops in Los Angeles, weeklong binges in some of the most dangerous crack houses in New York, and on and on. So now that I'm clean and healthy, I feel it's my duty to try to help the next person in line.

That's why I've become such an advocate for training, eating right, and getting the message out about how to live a healthier lifestyle. That's why I took up Ironman triathlons at forty-nine years of age, to challenge myself and to prove that this way of life works if you approach it properly. I also didn't wanna be one of those dudes who sit around in a bar talking shit like, "I used to be able to do this and that and blah blah fucking blah." Well, now I'm fifty-one and I'm doing four Ironmans this year. I'm also in the gym six days a week and still tour with my band, the Cro-Mags, getting down onstage like I did when I was twenty.

So, am I a little obsessive about training and eating right? Fuck yeah I am, but I'd rather be a fitness and health food addict than someone who's strung out on some type of drug or booze.

You have to start somewhere and that place is eliminating some of the bad shit. Start the work and use your body as a lab; it will tell you what you should and should not do. Usually with its help you'll make the right choices. Keep busy and keep the mind engaged in positive things and you will stay positive. That's why you also have to surround yourself with people who are on the same path. Don't be some negative fucker's drinking buddy, and, ladies, that goes for you as well. I don't know how many times I've heard some of my female friends tell me they wish they never went home with such-and-such a guy but they were drunk. Don't make bad choices, and if we are at all honest here, most bad choices are made when we are intoxicated.

Now let's take a look at that word for a second: *in-TOXIC-ated*. The root word being *toxic*, as in poisonous to your fucking body, numb-nuts. Maybe that's why when you drink you barf your brains out. That's the body's way of telling you, "Yo, jerk-off, this shit ain't supposed to be in here." The other thing most people do after a night of hard charging is to end up at some sleazebag all-night diner eating God knows what and going to sleep with a full stomach of all that poison rotting in their intestines. If you've been out all night drinking and eating toxins, do you really think you're going to get up in the morning and go to the gym, play hoops, do yoga, swim, bike, or run a 10K?

Let's be honest here, because my money's on a definitive *no* and if by some miracle you do make it, your performance will be total shit. Now, just imagine doing that year after year, partying away, eating bad food, and the rest that follows. Sooner or later there's going to be a breakdown in the machine. In other words, disease will strike.

Take the best example of the above-mentioned scenario if you will, these so-called rock stars. Oh yeah, nowadays with this microwave insta-fame culture we have, everybody dreams about becoming a rock star or celebrity overnight and partying like one, except they forgot to read the small print in their contract with the devil. The ones who they are trying to emulate have died, are dying, or are on their way to death. I've been playing music since the early eighties and from what I've seen, it ain't no dream.

DON'T SWEAT THE SMALL STUFF

Another thing that leads to bad health is stress. It's been medically proven that too much stress breaks down the body's immune system and leads to disease. Stress isn't just caused by some asshole that you want to choke the living shit out of (although that is a factor). It's also caused by eating bad food.

Follow me here while I break this down. See, our bodies all have a certain acidity level in the blood—referred to as the pH level. The scale of pH levels ranges from highly acidic (battery acid) to highly alkaline (soapy water), with plain old water right in the middle. The pH balance in your body is very important to overall health. If your body's pH is acidic—0 to 6 on the pH scale—most of the time, you are putting unnecessary stress on your immune and digestive systems. Your body also counteracts a high acidity level by releasing calcium from your bones to balance it—which is not good news for you or your bones.

Water has a pH balance of 7, which is neutral. A pH balance of 8 to 14 is considered alkaline. For optimum health you want to aim for a diet that is slightly alkaline, and lucky for you, that's just what a plant-based diet will help you do. You can buy pH test strips at any health food store—you just wet one with saliva and it will tell you where you are on the scale. If you have been eating a lot of acidic foods like meat, dairy, eggs, processed wheat, rice, and other crap, you probably have a very acidic pH level. You can bring your body back into balance by consuming high-alkaline foods like green juice, garlic, berries, oranges, bananas, kale, pumpkins, squash, peas, green tea, and most other fruits and vegetables. These will reduce the acid in your bloodstream and bring you back to the alkaline range.

And then there's the kind of stress that *does* come from some asshole you want to punch in the face. If you made the necessary dietary changes and still notice an acidic pH level, mental stress could be the culprit. You must monitor your mental stress level and utilize stress-reduction techniques like punching the shit out of a heavy bag instead of a person; going for a run; or doing a little yogic breathing. And never eat angry. Ever. If I'm stressed about something I wait until the feeling subsides before I eat. That's what my Italian ginzo friends call *agita*, and it's a killer on your digestive system. It's all about having the stress-management tools and techniques in your arsenal to help reduce stress both mentally and physically. Cutting down on stress will lead to a healthier life overall.

Let me give you an example of how much stress can impact your health. When I first stepped up my fitness training, I kinda bugged the shit out of my friend Brendan Brazier, who is a world-class triathlete, author, and plant-based lifestyle expert (more on him later). Luckily for me he's Canadian, eh, and one of the nicest dudes in the world. Anyway, I was noticing that I wasn't sleeping well at night, waking up fatigued and with very stiff muscles. I even gained some weight despite training for hours on end. That's when Brendan hipped me to the culprit: cortisol.

Cortisol is a hormone that the body releases when it's under stressful conditions from either diet or life. Things like eating shit food, partying, and mental stressors like dealing with all the new hipster assholes in New York. When stress goes up, cortisol goes up, and when cortisol is up, you can't enter the deepest stage of sleep, which is imperative for athletes to recover. When cortisol levels are down you sleep well; you wake up refreshed and ready to train again. Basically you're fully rejuvenated.

So what did I do to reverse the issue? Well, as Brendan told me and says in his book, *Thrive*, "You need to eat more 'net-gain-nutrition foods.'" In other words, I cut out all processed foods like tofu, wheat bread, and other processed stuff, because even though they're plant-based, they aren't the best fuel for an athlete. I did what he said. I swapped in unprocessed, whole-food, plant-based organic foods. Within a week I noticed the change. My cortisol dropped and I was sleeping well, waking up recovered and refreshed, and the weight came off. I also stayed away from the douche-bag hipsters or anyone else for that matter who pissed me the fuck off. Instead of cracking them I'd walk away breathing deeply and chanting, "I will not kick his ass, I will not kick his ass." As I said, avoidance of bad food and interactions with shitty people is the key to happiness.

I'll keep it short and sweet here because I think I made my point. Death is part of life. That is an undeniable truth, and it's not something that you can control. But how you live your life and the quality of it you get to enjoy while you're here—*that* you have control over. Me personally, I don't want to live in fantasyland, talking about the good old days and what I used to be able to do. Fuck that. I want to talk about what I'm doing and what I'm preparing to do. I finish a triathlon and sign up for the next one. You have to set goals and you have to smash the living shit out of them. And you can't do that when you're perpetually hungover or looking for your next fix.

To accomplish my goals I need to stay sober and stress-free as much as possible. Often when people get stressed, they falsely believe the answer is going out and getting fucked-up. That's the big lie. I can guarantee you with 100 percent certainty that when you come down off whatever it is you're high on, your problems will be multiplied. Drugs and booze only add fuel to the fire of negativity. They also lead to other bad choices. Bottom line, it's one big downward spiral.

So take control of your life by getting a handle on your stress and changing how you treat your body. This is science, and as in any science experiment, you start with a formula, you apply it, and you get a result. Don't alter the formula! Do what's in here and do all of it. Hands down you'll become one of the fittest badasses on two legs.

MEAT IS FOR PUSSIES

THE FIVE-LETTER CURSE WORD*

I want to take a brief moment to address something you might be wondering about as you read through this book. You will notice that there's a five-letter word I don't use when I'm talking about a meat-free diet. This particular word makes people cringe; it has come to have so many negative associations and stereotypes that I could fill another book on that subject alone. So was it merely by chance that I've failed to use it as I write this book? Hell no. It was a deliberate fucking move on my part and this section is the only place in the entire book that you will find me using this term.

Now, I myself am 100 percent "V-E-G-A-N," meaning I don't eat animal products, wear animal hides, or use or consume products containing animal by-products, nor do I support any industry that kills animals or tests on them. But I have been around this movement almost thirty-four years, and the truth is that too many of the people waving the V-flag are not people I wish to be lumped in with. And before the rest of you *vegan* people get your organic cotton panties in a bunch, let me explain myself so you don't write me off as some kind of a traitor.

---

* This message brought to you by the sane people who eat a plant-based diet.

I personally believe the negative connotations that have come to be associated with the V-word can be attributed to the judgmental, self-righteous attitudes of a particular subgroup of individuals. Case in point: when Jay-Z and Beyoncé announced in December 2013 that they were choosing to go on a twenty-two-day "plant-based" diet, the vegan haters came out of their little reclaimed wood wormholes and attacked. "Oh, they'll probably give up. They're just part-time vegan posers. Look, she's wearing a coat with fur on the collar . . ." And on and fucking on. Listen, douche bags, if everyone on the entire planet followed in their footsteps and did a twenty-two-day plant-based diet, we could start to solve a lot of big problems. So instead of criticizing, I give them props. Whether they stick with it or not, the fact is that they used their platform to get the word out about a plant-based diet and probably influenced millions of people to scramble to their computers to do a Google search on "plant-based diets."

Additionally, a lot of self-proclaimed V-words have a propensity to be on the . . . how shall I put this, on the fat and out-of-fucking-shape side. It comes as a result of eating too many doughnuts and muffins, and generally being lazy bastards who'd rather criticize meat-eaters than go to the gym or exercise.

So here's my deal on all of this. Eating gives me life.

But is not *my life*. It's part of the process of my evolution in consciousness.

I mean, have you ever been in a room with a bunch of preachy vegans? Holy shit, talk about a painful experience. All the fuck they ever talk about is food, food, and more food. Thus the running joke, "How do you find the vegan in the room? Don't worry, they will let you know." How many fucking conversations about dairy-free desserts, raw veggie pâté, and flax crackers can one stomach? I have literally been close to walking over to a buffet and smashing a tray of hummus over their fucking heads. I refer to this crowd as "macro-psychotics"—they turn off everyone as soon as they open their mouths. What these people don't get is that example is always better than precept. In other words, you can rant all you want about the benefits of going plant based, but the ones who you are looking to convert will always check out your attitude and the way you carry yourself. Just because you eat fucking tofu doesn't make you better than anyone else.

I think to a large degree that's why the vegan and vegetarian movements have failed in the past. But, like anything else, things evolve and thank God for that. Nowadays there are some very cool, very humble and badass men and women taking up the cause who are changing the way people think about going plant based.

Yes, the conversation about food choices is an important one, given how many people are getting sick because of our food supply. But rule number one—let's not forget the philosophy at the heart of a plant-based lifestyle, which is compassion for *all* beings, and that means humans included. You will not change anyone's heart if you agitate their mind with a condescending attitude. There are some preachy, judgmental vegans who attacked me for the title of this book. In my eyes I think whatever starts the conversation and shows positive results is a good thing. And have I ruffled a few feathers along the way? Sure. I've been doing this long before they ever showed up. I'll take all the criticism these jerk-offs want to throw my way if it means I can open a few eyes and change a few minds.

So bottom line to the V-crowd: Let's drink our green juice, eat our lentils, and then move the fuck on. Let's convert people by showing them by example what badass motherfuckers they can be on a plant-based regime, and leave the judgment at the door.

CHAPTER **3**

THE GREAT

FOOD
BAMBOOZLE

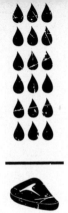

THE GREAT FOOD BAMBOOZLE

bam·boo·zle: to deceive by underhanded methods: dupe, hoodwink

I'm gonna be blunt. Your average American doesn't know shit about the crap he's stuffing in his face, and he's obsessed with it. How obsessed? A while back I was on the road in the deep South touring with my band and we got lost, so we pulled up at a light and asked your standard American couple down in them there parts (both were easily over three hundred pounds) for directions to the highway. So the husband leans out the driver's window and proceeds to help me out. "Okay, now you go down a half mile or so and take a left at the Wing-ding Sallies, the best dang fried chicken in the South in my opinion, go two more lights and there'll be a Pancake House on your right, if you hurry you can still make the $3.99 breakfast special and let me tell ya they got these little buttermilk cheese biscuits, man oh man, I can eat me a dozen of them things, anyway, make yourself another left, go about four lights, and you'll see a Burger King, don't turn there, go past it till you see the KFC, then take your right and when you pass the Steak-n-Shake the entrance to the highway is right there. Lord Jesus, I'll you what, all this damn talking made me hungry." And so before I could even thank him, off they went, tires screeching.

Now, just so you don't think I'm coming off with some holier-than-thou New York City attitude here, let me tell you something: I too was once obsessed with, even addicted to, food. I grew up in a bad foster home, being starved. I had to survive off the foster mother's Oreo spit sandwiches, Milk Bone dog biscuits (which I literally had to steal out of their dogs' mouths), rotten, mold-covered cold-cut sandwiches, and powdered milk loaded with white sugar. When I finally did reach adulthood and was able to provide for myself, I ate every fucking thing in sight and I ate it until my stomach was about to burst. The truth is, if I didn't change the way I ate I'd be tipping the scales at over three hundred pounds my damn self.

Food has been a battle my entire life, and the only way I was able to start winning was with the power of knowledge. I had to learn the facts and then more importantly apply what I had learned. I became like a sponge soaking it all up, writing it all down. I knew I had to beat this thing and the only way to do that was by getting informed about where my food came from.

And the same goes for you. Some of the things you'll read in this book may blow your mind or gross you out. It might make you angry to discover that there are companies out there that have a stake in keeping you fat, sick, and nearly dead. I just hope for your sake that you can channel that anger into the energy to make positive changes.

Watching the evening news recently, I conducted an experiment, as I often do at 6 p.m., just to gauge the programming being fed out to the masses. As I flipped through the channels during the commercial break, what did I see? Practically every other ad was either for erectile-dysfunction boner pills like Cialis (two channels ran it simultaneously) or other meds to control high cholesterol, acid reflux, or diabetes. And the list of side effects for one drug was actually a bit comedic. "Side effects may include: stroke, heart attack, vaginal dryness, trouble urinating, shortness of breath, diarrhea, sleepwalking, violent dreams, seizures, irritability, suicidal thoughts, depression, and death"! WTF, dude, all I had was a little skin rash.

So how the hell did America go from being a nation of fit, kick-ass fuckers to having the distinguished title of being one of the most obese, overmedicated, and sick nations on earth? I would argue that it's due in part to slick marketing (some call it brainwashing). That's why the first thing you have to do is erase everything from your memory banks in terms of the way you look at food and nutrition. Because beneath the surface of what you've been told by TV, the radio, even the government, there is something sinister and diabolical going on. Simply put, we have been bamboozled.

You see, my friends, most of the food on supermarket shelves these days did not exist a hundred years ago, and interestingly enough, there was no such thing as an obesity crisis then, either. Your food has undergone radical changes. A lot of what you find in the grocery store today has been genetically modified (more on that in a bit), is coated with toxic pesticides and chemical residue, has been injected with shit like rBGH (recumbent bovine growth hormone, a drug used to treat cattle that is illegal in many countries around the world),[7] and is loaded with hydrogenated oils, sugar, salt, and preservatives. In other words it's a bunch of chemical shit that I wouldn't feed to a fucking flea-infested homeless dog with mange in a slum in India.

Over the past fifty years we have become a nation of fat, lazy bastards whose days and nights are filled with sitting at a desk job, being glued in front of the TV, surfing the Internet, or playing video games for hours on end—all the while stuffing our faces with crap. And a note to all of you Call of Duty war gamers: you ain't a Special Forces operator and your online fantasy SEAL team doesn't need you tonight, as I have yet to ever meet a Navy SEAL with a gut the size of Maryland, a bottle of Ex-Lax, a jar of Tums, a year's supply of Doritos, a half gallon of Mountain Dew, and a COPD inhaler.

So let's backtrack for a moment to where all this insanity started, the dawn of the industrial revolution. Now, sure, there have been technological achievements in the last hundred or so years that have greatly benefited humanity, and not just with our food. But this so-called modern advancement has brought with it a slew of problems, particularly as we've moved away from eating locally grown, natural foods to chemically treated crops that require millions of tons of pesticides, herbicides, and fungicides to produce—and then are shipped to us from hundreds of miles away.[8] So you take that food and then process the shit out of it and add in a bunch more chemicals—artificial colors, preservatives, you name it—and you've got a country of fat, sick, prescription-drug-dependent people.

Some of the most brilliant minds in health and nutrition predict that if we continue on the path we are currently treading, today's generation of kids may be the first in the history of the planet to have a shorter life span than their parents.[9] Seriously, think about that. I'm already seeing how that can be true. Twelve-year-olds weighing in excess of 250 pounds, suffering from type 2 diabetes and coronary disease. These poor kids have already become addicted to crap. The food additives as well as the hyper-stimulating amounts of sugar, fat, and salt in processed foods have them coming back like crackheads fiending for a fix.

You think fast food isn't addictive? Watch the documentary film my friend Morgan Spurlock made, *Super Size Me*, where Morgan got the shakes when he detoxed off Mc-Donald's, just like a junkie coming off heroin. Or perhaps you caught the infamous "Chicken Nugget Beat Down Episode" on YouTube, where a woman pulled up at a Mc-Donald's drive-through one morning while the breakfast menu was still being served and tried to order the twelve-piece of chicken nuggets. When the woman working inside informed her it wasn't lunchtime yet, the chick got out of her car, punched the woman in the face, then dragged her through the takeout window screaming, "Bitch, I told you, I want my motherfuckin' nuggets!"

Now, I never laugh at another's expense, but I do feel that making a point through comedy is always better than standing on a soapbox. My mission is to make you take inventory of what you're stocking on your shelves and stuffing in your mouth, and if I can get you to laugh at the absurdity of what's going on, I'm all for it.

So how do we take back control of our health and stop

being our own worst enemy? Through the power of knowledge, and the first step in gaining that knowledge is to accept the fact that we don't know it all. And that's because we're not being given the facts by the people in charge of producing, regulating, and marketing our food.

Here's a little story for you from my daily life in New York City. I lent this book to my friend Pete, who is a pretty kick-ass fighter from the Netherlands. Then it was the holidays and I didn't see him for a while. When I finally did bump into him at the gym he came up to me and said, "First off, fuck you. Second, thank you." Please allow me to elaborate. He went on to explain that after reading the book, he was walking through the supermarket one day and quickly grabbed one of his favorite food items off the shelf. You know the kind—packaged so wonderfully, and, like a smiling politician, completely full of shit. Then something clicked in his brain—he remembered what he'd learned and stopped short before tossing it in his cart. He read the nutrition label. Then he put it back onto the shelf.

The information contained in this book instilled in him what I refer to as the "Stop and Think Mechanism." In other words, the ability to stop and ask yourself *what is this, where does it come from, and should I be eating it?* SATM is a marketing person's worst nightmare because it engages your intelligence to make the right choice, not the easy choice. So he cursed me because he couldn't eat his packaged poison, but ultimately he thanked me because of the positive changes he's experienced and the knowledge he's gained.

KNOWLEDGE GOES A LONG WAY

I've laid out this chapter to be a wake-up call and it needs to be. The food manufacturers and pharmaceutical companies don't care if you get sick—and in fact it is in their best interest if you do. People are conspiring against our health for profit—a profit that topped an incredible $340 billion in 2011.[10] Think I'm a conspiracy theorist? Let me throw some facts your way. Did you know that the clinical trials run to demonstrate the safety of drugs to the Food and Drug Administration (FDA) are conducted by the drug companies themselves? So the food companies are pumping our food full of toxic shit under the lazy eye of the FDA, and the drug companies are enabling us to keep eating their poison by treating us with the drugs that aren't actually tested by the government. Doesn't seem like a coincidence to me.

And boy do they have some racket going. You rub some toxic shit all over yourself, spray cleaning chemicals in your home, go eat your drug-infected hamburger on some processed white bread with a list of ingredients as long as a porn star's dick, wash it down with a liter of Coca-Cola, and the next thing you know the dudes in the white coats are breaking out their notepads and prescribing pills for you and your family. We are at war, people: the war to take back our health.

We all have the potential for infinite greatness in this life—and the right to health and happiness. That's not some new-age bullshit; that's the truth. As I mentioned, I have not had an easy life. I've been shot, stabbed, robbed, and beat down and I've had to return the favor in more than a few instances. I spent years in juvenile lockups. Before I changed, trust me, I was someone you definitely did not want to bump into in a dark alley.

If people like me can change, there's hope for everyone. And the first step for me was to give up meat and the rest of the poisons I was ingesting. When I did that, something clicked inside. From there a whole new awareness and perspective opened up, new doors, new paths. I challenge you to do the same. I will give you the tools. If you use them, I can guarantee you that crazy, beautiful things will happen in your life.

The nineteenth-century philosopher Arthur Schopenhauer said truth passes through three phases:

FIRST, it is ridiculed.
SECOND, it is fiercely and violently opposed.
THIRD, it becomes self-evident.

So maybe right now you're thinking, "What's this idiot talking about? What a bunch of bullshit." Then you might get pissed off. "Who the fuck is this asshole to tell me anything? Fuck him!" Finally, as you let go and remember to stay open to learning new things, you might even try to make a few changes to your lifestyle and then . . . voilà! There's a truckload of truth waiting for you.

This is a process that takes time. But it's worth the investment—I am living proof, as are people like Fred Bisci, who wrote the afterword to this book. At eighty-four Fred still runs daily and has more energy than most people half his age. How? He has a great saying: "Any doubt, leave it out." And what he means is, if you encounter food and you don't know how it was produced or recognize its ingredients, don't eat it. Bottom line: the only food you should be eating is food that's found in nature, not a factory. Don't let the bamboozlers bamboozle you.

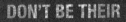

DON'T BE THEIR

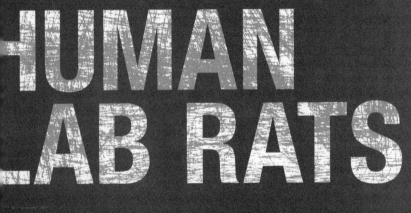

HUMAN
LAB RATS

CHAPTER 4

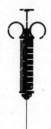

DON'T BE THEIR HUMAN LAB RATS

A lot of dudes I talk to have never heard of a GMO. Yet they are probably eating them every day. That's because GMOs (genetically modified organisms) make up a huge part of our food supply. To be exact: 88 percent of corn, 90 percent of canola, 95 percent of sugar beets, and 93 percent of soy produced in the United States is grown from genetically modified seeds. If you're thinking, "I don't eat beets or corn!"—think again, buddy. The by-products of these crops can be found in just about every processed food on the shelf. Seriously, read some product labels and see for yourself just how many contain soy or canola oil, lecithin, sugar, high-fructose corn syrup (the latter two come from sugar beets), and so on. You'd be shocked. Packaged foods are also loaded with GMO soy in the form of hydrogenated oils, lecithin, emulsifiers, tocopherol (a vitamin E supplement), and proteins. That being the case, don't you think it might be a good idea for you to learn what the hell a GMO is—and to be given a heads-up when you're putting one in your body?

Well, I can give you the knowledge about what GMOs are, but unfortunately our friends at the FDA don't seem to think you need to know whether or not they're in your food—because they don't require foods containing GMO crops to be labeled as such. As a matter of fact the FDA chose to ignore a petition with one million signatures calling for the mandatory labeling of all GMOs in America.[11]

To begin to understand why this is dangerous, let's take a closer look at what a GMO is. A GMO is an organism whose DNA has been altered using genetic engineering techniques. When you transfer new DNA into foods it allows them to acquire modified traits: improved shelf life, greater resistance to pests, the ability to withstand harsh environmental conditions. Bottom line: scientists create jacked-up Frankencrops that have the ability to thrive under harsh conditions.

Now, you might be thinking, "Hey, man, what's wrong with that? I mean, shit, if plants don't get destroyed they can feed more people, right?" Well, first glances are usually deceptive, so just as with any good investigation let's peel back that shiny outer coat and dig a little deeper.

There is a lot of debate about the safety of GMOs—you will see articles written by "scientists" on both sides of the aisle, though the fact is, most of the good press you see for GMOs is backed by scientists who work for Monsanto, the country's largest producer of genetically modified seeds (as well as manufacturing the commercially marketed pesticide Roundup and, in the not so recent past, DDT, PCBs, Agent Orange, and rBGH). But if you're looking for an unbiased opinion, how about the American Academy of Environmental Medicine, a group composed mostly of traditionally trained physicians? Here's what they've said on the matter: "There's so much evidence of harm from animal feeding studies [GMO crops are fed to livestock] including reproductive disorders, immune system problems, accelerated aging and more."[12] And data from our very own U.S. Department of Agriculture says that over the first thirteen years of commercial use of GMO crops (1996–2008), herbicide use in the United States increased by 383 million pounds.[13]

Now, I have to admit I never really paid much attention to this issue because I eat mostly unprocessed, organic whole food. But then, as it turns out, I too was unknowingly consuming GMOs because I was also eating some packaged goods that were not clearly labeled. So being the pain in the ass that I am, I called the number listed on one of the boxes, and to my surprise, I found out my food contained GMOs.

Biotech companies like Monsanto have lobbied furiously against having to label their food as such. Why? Here's one of Monsanto's responses: "Requiring labeling for ingredients that do not pose a health issue would undermine both our labeling laws and consumer confidence." Huh. So if GMOs are safe, why *not* label them? I wonder if it might have something to do with fearing potential lawsuits down the road?

The funny thing is that when it comes to consumer confidence, I guess they're right—studies show that nine out of ten Americans want GMOs to be clearly labeled on their food, and say that they would definitely avoid them if they were labeled. And a recent Nielsen poll named "non-GMO" as the fastest-growing new label for store brands.

FUCK YOU VERY MUCH, MONSANTO

Do me a favor and google "the most evil company on the planet" and see what name pops up. Go ahead, I'll wait.

Right—now you understand my sentiments above. Monsanto has a long history of making things that are bad for people, and not disclosing the dangers of its toxic products to the public. For example, Monsanto was the only American company to produce the highly toxic man-made chemical polychlorinated biphenyls, better known as PCBs, which are used in some plastics. Once PCBs enter an animal or human body they are absorbed within fat cells and stay there. This then causes the PCB to build up and produces a chain reaction that contaminates land and wildlife—a process known as bioaccumulation.

A horrific example was made of the people of Anniston, Alabama, when the Monsanto factory hid PCB toxins in wetlands and polluted a nearby creek.[14] The contamination was so devastating that when scientists released fish into the creek to test toxicity, the majority died in three and a half minutes. And that was just the wildlife—think about the soil and the contamination caused by this non-biodegradable chemical that will linger in our environment forever. Listen, people, if you think the devil resides in hell, I got news for you: he's sitting in Creve Coeur, Missouri,* cheering them on.

The same rings true for GMOs. Once *they* are released into the wild there's no way to control them. The harsh chemicals farmers use on these biocrops contaminate every other field around the area, and they ruin organically grown crops on other farms when the wind carries their pollen or seeds to far-flung destinations. And by the way,

---

* Monsanto is headquartered in Creve Coeur, Missouri.

if Monsanto's seeds *do* cross-pollinate with other farmers' crops, Monsanto steps in and claims copyright infringement, because for the first time in the history of our planet, a company has been allowed to own a patent on organic life. So what does Monsanto do? Sue the farmers and make them destroy their crops and seeds.

Monsanto has also found a way into your favorite dairy products by injecting milk cows with recombinant bovine growth hormone (rBGH), marketed as Posilac. Of course, if it's injected into a cow, it's also being injected into every product produced from that cow's milk. So rBGH isn't just bad news for that poor, abused cow—it's bad news for all of you who eat cheese and ice cream. Recent research has linked dairy foods produced with Monsanto's rBGH to breast and prostate cancers.

Do me a favor—sit back for a second and give all this some thought. Why are we letting companies whose main business is the manufacturing and selling of toxic pesticides and genetically modified seeds produce our food and develop crops that are dependent on their own chemicals? I mean, can't we see through the game they're running? No one should be allowed to create a monopoly on our food chain—especially one that threatens our health.

So how do they get away with pushing their products on us, the unsuspecting public? Some people (me) would suggest that Monsanto gets help from very high places in the U.S. government. Talk about letting the fox in the henhouse. You would think there would have been outrage and demonstrations against the growing power and global control that Monsanto is attaining, right? Well, there have been some, but Monsanto is so well protected by the government that protests haven't made much of a dent in the problem. We can't continue to let this go on. Many European countries have completely banned GMOs. What the hell is wrong with us in America?

Here are the weapons we need to fight this with: knowledge and money.

Let's start with the first one. Not all GMO food is labeled as such, but there is a way to learn the source of your produce, even without forthright labeling: the bar code. You know those little stickers you see on fruits and vegetables at the grocery store? They actually serve a purpose, they aint't just there for shits and giggles. They mean something. The first number on the bar code tells you all you need to know about the source of your food. Here is the rundown:

IGNORE the 4—it means conventional pesticides and dyes are used and it may be genetically modified
HATE the 8—it is GMO and a no-go
DINE on the 9—it's organically produced.

You can also follow the advice of Jeffrey Smith's Non-GMO Shopping Guide, at www.nongmoshoppingguide.com.

Action number two: support organic farming. We're the consumers, and if we use our buying power to support local, organic, responsibly produced food, eventually big business will listen. Remember, we vote three times a day with our wallets and purses. Every meal is an opportunity to support the people who produce our foods without chemicals.

Okay, and maybe there's a third weapon: advocacy. Demand from your political representatives that all GMO food be labeled as such. This isn't just a political issue—this is about your personal health and the future of food. This GMO scam could potentially be the biggest hoax ever conducted on the American people. Monsanto has even threatened lawsuits against states like Vermont if they pass laws that require labels on genetically engineered food and ban the routine industry practice of labeling GMO-tainted foods as "natural" or "all natural." These guys are like the neighborhood bullies that somebody needs to step up to and beat the living shit out of. That somebody is us. We can do it by spreading this knowledge and boycotting their products.

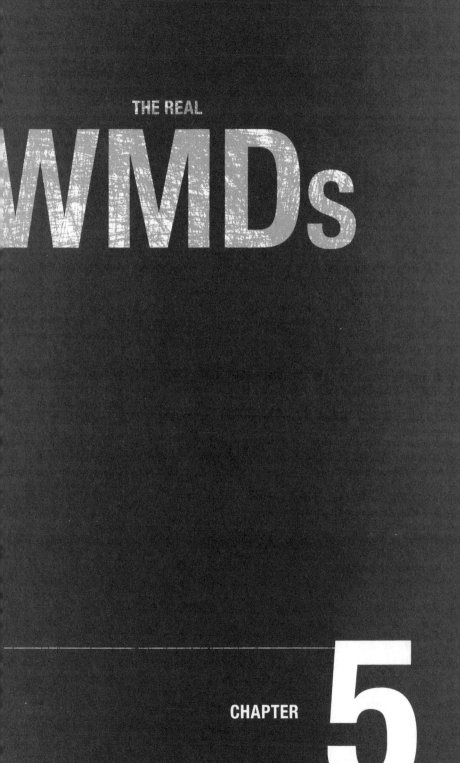

THE REAL

WMDs

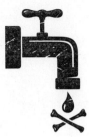

CHAPTER 5

THE REAL WMDs

A Fight for Our Lives

Lately it seems like most people are in a semi-constant state of panic over the economy. It's even replaced the preoccupation with and fear of terrorism for the most part, hasn't it? So we tighten our belts for a while—we Americans are a resilient bunch, we'll get through it and survive. What I would like to understand is why the health epidemic, the disease crisis in America, isn't generating the same amount of fear and anxiety. I mean, shit, food is killing more people than terrorists, and yet I still see people sitting outside BBQ restaurants eating an enormous friggin' pile of smoked meat and washing it down with a quart-sized electric-blue drink.

I recently had a conversation with someone about this exact issue and his point went something like this: "Yo, my man, I know this shit's probably gonna make my ass sick, but they got medication for that. When it's my time, it's my time; while I'm here I wanna enjoy myself." First of all, how much could this dude really be enjoying himself? He was severely overweight, had problems in the toilet department (he told me on that particular day he was backed up worse than a brotha at a chitlin-eating contest), was always fatigued, suffered depression, hadn't got laid in months, and had the warning signs of type 2 diabetes. Second, I can tell you personally, having spent time in a cancer ward, where people actually are confronting the fact that they may die, that that kind of attitude does not stand up to reality. No one wants to die, believe me.

Albert Einstein said the definition of insanity is doing the same thing over and over again and expecting a different result. Well, another type of insanity is to keep doing things over and over again *that you know are making you sick*, but you just add medications to cover up symptoms and prolong the inevitable.

The reality is that we need to focus on prevention, not treatment. All drugs can do is treat the symptoms and, yes, that may be great for the pharmaceutical companies, but where does that leave us? So, sure, we are getting screwed over for profit, but we are screwing ourselves and causing this health crisis by living these poisonous, lazy lifestyles. That, my friends, we have control over, and even though there are many forces conspiring against us, I say a little accountability is in order on our end for what we are doing to ourselves. Our lives have become a big, toxic puzzle—and when you piece together the food, chemicals, and medications being shoved down our throats with our own bad habits and choices, we can start to get a clear picture of our overall health.

Now, for anyone who has been living under a rock, WMD stands for "weapon of mass destruction"—and while Americans were led to believe they were being created in Iraq, the truth is that they're closer than you think. All you have to do is open your refrigerator or cupboard or medicine cabinet and take a gander at what the hell you're ingesting and putting on your body. I mean, seriously, give it some thought. The way we live every day is devastating our lives, our children's lives, and the planet—yet we stand frozen with fear every time we hear bad news about the stock market or see that same old al-Qaeda training film on Fox News. My message to the boogeymen screaming, "Death to America!"? Don't worry, dudes, we're doing a pretty good damn job of killing ourselves without your help.

WMD might as well stand for "weapon of mass deception," too, since the companies that are selling this toxic shit don't exactly print how deadly their product is on the package or show photos of sick people on the label. Like those anti-cigarette commercials where people are wheezing and talking through a voice box with a tracheotomy— they're pretty effective, right? Imagine if there was a photo on the side of every Chef Boyardee can, McDonald's burger wrapper, or Oscar Mayer lunch meat package, showing an obese person having his colon removed or getting open-heart surgery. Maybe even a pic of a diabetic getting a gangrenous foot cut off on a 64-ounce 7-Eleven Slurpee cup? That wouldn't exactly go over big in the sales department, would it?

STOP THE CHEMICAL WARFARE

Now, let's talk for a minute here about why these WMDs are so dangerous. Have you ever heard of free radicals? No, they're not the dudes who just got out of jail after an Occupy Wall Street rally. Free radicals are molecules in our cells that are "unstable" because they're missing a few electrons—and so they seek out other molecules to attach themselves to in order to increase their stability. They are produced naturally, and also when the body is subjected to toxins. When free radicals bond to other molecules in the body, they can cause damage to cells or to DNA contained within the cells. Free radicals are thought to play a part in the aging process, in some autoimmune diseases, and in the development of cancer. Excessive free radicals have the potential to do damage in your cells that harms your DNA—which literally contains your genetic blueprint—and results in cells mutating into cancerous cells.[15] Every chemical and toxin in your body fuels the creation of free radicals. Processed foods generate more free radicals than whole foods, and have fewer vitamins and minerals to counteract their effects. On top of this, more than seventy thousand chemicals are used regularly, and chronic exposure to some of them can give you cancer.[16]

So that brings up the question of the day: If you knew all of this, would you change your daily habits? I'd like to think most people would, especially those suffering from disease, or those who have lost loved ones from it, because sadly enough sometimes it takes a terrible tragedy to wake us up. But how angry would you become if you found out that the people selling toxic food and other products knew exactly how dangerous their stuff was before they poisoned your loved ones with it? Well, I hope you'd get really pissed, because that's exactly what's going down.

The good news is, we can take a proactive stance in fighting disease by avoiding these products and by eating a plant-based diet rich in antioxidants and chlorophyll foods, both of which destroy free radicals.[17] Do not procrastinate. You needed to start this yesterday.

OUR KIDS ARE WORTH FIGHTING FOR

I want to take a brief moment here to talk about the impact of these WMDs on our future—and children are our future. I believe as so many others do that the soaring rise of childhood diseases can be directly correlated to our modern diet and lifestyle. According to the U.S. Centers for Disease Control and Prevention, a staggering 1 in 88 kids in America is now diagnosed with autism.[18] Other studies show that almost everyone over age ten has fatty streaks in their arteries, an early sign of heart disease.[19] One in three children born in the United States will develop type 2 diabetes.[20] And approximately 10 percent of American children ages four to five are overweight, double the number of overweight kids twenty years ago.[21] We are breeding a country of very sick people, and it all starts with our kids.

For starters, let's look at how we feed our kids in school. The National School Lunch Program subsidizes low-cost lunches for public school students, and if you look at what they're serving, it's loaded with toxins: pesticide-treated fresh or preservative-filled canned fruits and veggies; dairy and meat that may contain hormones and antibiotics; and processed grains devoid of nutrient value. That's pure insanity. And people wonder why their kids seem to be getting sick all the time?

The school lunch program is another WMD, and the meat and dairy industries are making hundreds of millions of dollars a year serving our kids this crap. But it goes on because of lax government standards and loopholes—like when food manufacturers are able to claim pizza meets FDA approval as a serving of vegetables, or because the Department of Agriculture recommends that children over nine should drink three cups of milk daily (that's a pound and a half of milk a day). This all sucks for our kids, but, hey, it's great for the vampires from Big Pharma waiting in the wings who know these kids are going to be on some type of drug for the rest of their lives. Your children are being handed poisoned foods at every step of their young lives, and the repercussions of that are borne out by the statistics and our own two eyes.

What's going on in this country sickens me, especially when I see those commercials for St. Jude Children's Hospital. The pain and suffering of those kids and their parents piss me the hell off, but also inspire me to get the word out. We all have the right to lead healthy lives. We have the right to be informed about the dangers of the products we purchase for ourselves and our families. Victor Hugo said, "There's nothing more powerful than an idea whose time has come." Well, my fellow earthlings, that time is now.

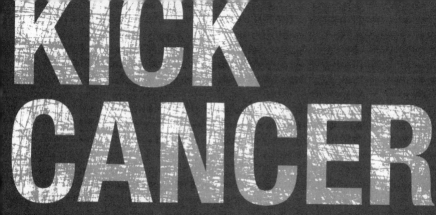

KICK CANCER

(AND OTHER DISEASES)

(AND OTHER DISEASES)

IN THE NUTS

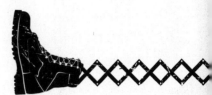

KICK CANCER (AND OTHER DISEASES) IN THE NUTS

It seems like cancer—its victims, treatments, experiments, and drugs—makes headlines every day. These bullshit stories go a little something like this: "In a sad piece of news, Fred Shapiro died at the age of fifty-two after a five-year bout with pancreatic cancer. Although the cancer had recently gone into remission, things took a turn for the worse in recent months. Thankfully, a groundbreaking drug is awaiting approval by the FDA to cure this form of cancer and should be available to the public soon."

Not once have I heard what anyone was eating before they got cancer or what they were eating after it went into remission and came back. I'm sure we all know a friend, relative, or loved one who has become afflicted with some form of cancer. It's a complicated disease, for sure, with a lot of different risk factors. But the truth is that the further away we get from nature and eating the plants nature provides for us, the more we delve into an artificial life of TV, video games, computers, chemicals, preservatives, and meat carcasses rotting in our intestines, the more susceptible we become to diseases like cancer.

I want you to be able to enjoy every single day of your life. So even if you're some twenty-five-year-old hotshot who eats whatever the fuck you want, you had better start paying attention to your diet while you're still young. Cancer and other diseases are our bodies' way of telling us that something is wrong. Your lifestyle and your genetics all factor into your risk profile, but the knockout punch—and the one you have control over—is the horrendous, rotting, chemical-laden food you're consuming.

A CLOSER LOOK

So let's look at what we willingly put in our bodies and how that impacts our cancer risk. Well, for one thing, consuming red meat such as beef, pork, lamb, and processed meat has been linked to colorectal cancer. A 2005 study of almost 130,000 people between the ages of fifty and seventy-four showed that a high consumption of red and processed meats was linked with a substantial increase in the risk of cancer in the colon and rectum. Based on that evidence, the *Harvard Medical School Family Health Guide* offers this guidance: "the evidence suggests that you'd be wise to limit your consumption [of red and processed meats]."[22] Eating nitrate-filled processed meats—things like deli meat, sausage, and salami—has been associated with an increased risk of dying from cancer and heart disease.[23] Want more? A 2012 analysis of all the best studies out there shows that vegetarians have significantly lower cancer rates than carnivores.[24]

Rather than focus on the carcinogens we willingly ingest or expose ourselves to every day, however, most doctors are focused only on the diagnosis and treatment. In a book by Drs. W. John Diamond and W. Lee Cowden, *Cancer Diagnosis: What to Do Next*, Burton Goldberg, renowned voice of holistic medicine, relates a story to this effect: "A man was diagnosed with prostate cancer and his tumor biopsy was examined by two types of doctors: a pathologist and a toxicologist. The pathologist saw only clear signs of cancer in the tissue sample, but the toxicologist found something more because she knew what to look for. She found abnormally high levels of a variety of carcinogenic chemicals including arsenic, chlordane and DDT. In other words, there was evidence of pesticides and other environmental toxins in the tissue sample itself. Most conventional oncologists disregard toxicity as a factor in cancer. The patient was overloaded with toxins and his liver could no longer detoxify his body. With this gap in understanding, the treatment he designed for the patient couldn't possibly be effective, because it would fail to address the root cause."

THE ROOT CAUSE. To get to the root cause of illness we need to ask, *Why* are we sick? You can treat the cancer by pumping dangerous chemicals into the body, but if you don't get to the root cause, you will just keep getting sick and keep getting treated with the same drugs. It's sad to see how prostate cancer is booming in America. No heterosexual dude likes anyone putting a finger in his ass; but if you contract this cancer, they'll be putting a lot more than that up there. If that doesn't sound too appealing to all of you drive-through junkies, I suggest you pay close attention: studies have shown that exposure to heterocyclic amines (HCAs) and polycyclic aromatic hydrocarbons (PAHs) from meat cooked at high temperatures can cause cancer in animals.[25] And eating large amounts of brightly colored fruits and vegetables (yellow, orange, red, green, white, blue, purple), whole grains, and beans may decrease the risk of developing certain cancers as well as diabetes, hypertension, and heart disease.[26]

If you do what I have done, and that is to look at the

toxic load we are being subjected to on a daily basis, it will blow your fucking mind. It's no wonder our immune systems have been compromised and that we are becoming more and more diseased, thanks to everything from the next level of deadly pesticides being sprayed on our fruits and veggies; hormones and other drugs in our meat; pollutants in our water, air, and land from chemical companies and industrial farming operations; dangerous shit in our personal hygiene products like shampoo, deodorant, makeup, and diapers; and home cleaning products and furniture laced with plastics and fire-retardant chemicals. You owe it to yourself and your loved ones, especially children with developing immune systems, to take a deeper look at every single thing you use in your daily lives and investigate what the fuck's in it.

THE BIG C AND THE BIG LIES

Ignorance is not bliss, people. Having knowledge that explains why we're becoming sick is the first step in the healing process; only then can we prevent disease from happening at all. Modern medicine is losing the battle against cancer. They keep promising us that one day they will find a way to annihilate cancer from the face of the earth. It's like a million-dollar check you won't ever be able to cash. Don't believe the lies. According to the National Cancer Institute, cancer is the second leading cause of death by disease between infancy and fifteen years of age.[27] Sure, they've made some progress, but the idea that we will one day have a "cure," despite the billions being poured into drug research, seems far-fetched to me. The "cure" is to dramatically reduce our chances of developing cancer at all by leading nontoxic lives. Don't you think your children deserve a long, healthy life—a life free from suffering? And don't you want to be around to see your kids graduate from college, get married, and give you some grandchildren?

Change what you eat and the way you live your life today. And if you're ever diagnosed with cancer, I would encourage you to explore your treatment options before you suffer through dangerous (and dangerously expensive) chemo chemicals and radiation treatments. I'll never forget what it was like to watch my mother's boyfriend, Carl, suffer through horrible side effects of cancer treatments at the end of his life. The guy was so miserable he just gave up mentally, physically, and spiritually. It's worth knowing about what else is out there, and asking your doctor lots of questions. Your life is too valuable not to do so.

HEALTH IS WEALTH

_____

I admit I am a layperson when it comes to medical stuff, but I have been investigating alternative health treatments for a long time now. I've attended seminars by Viktoras P. Kulvinskas (author of *Survival into the 21st Century*) and other Hippocrates Health Institute advocates as far back as 1981. I listened to cassette recordings of renowned alternative medicine advocate Gary Null doing his radio show on WBAI in New York City more than twenty years ago. I used to listen to him on a small radio I had in my burnt-out squat before anyone knew who the hell he was. I even took notes . . . by candlelight!

Why? Because everything they said about why people get sick opened my eyes. What we're putting in our bodies and *not* putting in our bodies plays a huge role in our health. Be inspired to heal and get healthy. Living in this material world means we have to suffer birth, old age, and death, but the amount of disease we suffer is largely up to us.

You want to get scared straight? Go visit a cancer ward and talk to the patients there. After seeing Carl in the hospital as he was near death, and after taking a look at the other cancer patients on his floor, I will never take my health for granted again.

LIVE LONG AND PROSPER

———————

Everyone wants to live a long, healthy, and active life . . . right? Hell yeah you do. But the truth is that most guys care more about their 401(k)s, stocks, bonds, or cars than they do about their health. Well, if you're not healthy enough to live a normal life, who the fuck cares about how much money you've got or what kind of car you drive? I mean, don't the out-of-shape fuckers in the Porsches, Ferraris, and Corvettes just crack you up? Dude, that young, hot chick may hang with you for some free trips and presents, but she'll leave you in a New York minute for a fit dude driving a beat-up '74 Dodge Dart.

Health is wealth. It's *true*. Hell, I'm fifty-one and all the guys who made fun of me back in 1981 for the way I decided to live my life are coming to me for health advice now. Then there's the other dudes I run into, who feed me a bullshit line that goes something like, "Dude, my grandfather ate meat, smoked, and drank vodka his entire life and still lived to be a hundred and three." Well, not to diss Gramps, but he's the exception to the rule. First of all, we're living in much different times. Most of the meat we're eating nowadays is mass-produced and injected with hormones and toxic drugs. But it's not just meat; this is the worst time in the history of this planet to be eating fish, eggs, or dairy. Frankly, I'm amazed you guys aren't grow-ing a third nut . . . or are you? Take a quick break to check.

Second, it's a quality-of-life issue. Sure, you can live for a long time on a shitty diet—just make sure there's a forklift in your house to get you up the stairs and a motor scooter in your driveway to get you to your mailbox. I know people who live their lives like that. These nimrods nearly have an asthma attack every time they scale one flight of stairs. I saw one pudged-out, alcohol-drinking, meat-eating, chain-smoking fucker in a three-thousand-dollar custom suit and the guy couldn't even tie his thousand-dollar shoes without oxygen. On top of that, he hadn't seen his dick in six years.

Look at the guys who got hip to the organic veggie life-style early on. Dudes like Jack LaLanne, Paul Bragg, Fred Bisci, and many others who remained active well into their sixties, seventies, and even their eighties. At eighty-five, the Juiceman Jay Kordich was still boning his young, hot wife. And, personally speaking, if I want to bike a hundred miles, run a marathon, take a two-mile swim, box, wrestle, dance for hours, perform onstage with an all-out mosh-pit assault, do backflips, and then go kick it with my lady after . . . I can. See, I made the investment in my health, and as your bro I urge you to do the same. Just take it one day at a time and this investment will pay huge dividends. You may say, "Ahhh, I ain't got the time." But remember: the same people who used that bullshit excuse with me thirty years ago are now getting their cancerous colons removed, having their bodies ravaged by diabetes, undergoing open-heart surgery, and suffering from the ultimate manhood killer. If they had just listened, their dicks wouldn't have been served a death sentence. It all comes back to that old Benjamin Franklin quote: "An ounce of prevention is worth a pound of cure." Right on, Benny.

The best thing about the future is that it comes one day at a time, so implement changes little by little. Examine your diet and keep track of the toxins you ingest and the stressful situations you encounter. Ask yourself, "How can I improve my immune system?" It doesn't make you a pussy to care about yourself and others. The bottom line is that life is better when you're healthy. So seize the day and seize control of your life.

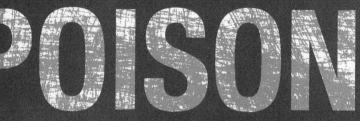

GET THE

POISON
OUT

CHAPTER 7

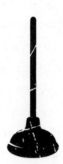

GET THE POISON OUT

First thing's first: you need to change what you're putting into your body, because most of it is poison. Think about your body like a mini-earth. Just as water flows through the oceans and rivers, you have blood that flows throughout your body via veins, arteries, and capillaries. Like the earth's core, you have organs, muscles, tissues, and fibers that hold everything together. Pollute any of these and you're in trouble. So let's start with the place where the shit you eat does the most damage: the colon.

> **NOTE:** If you have a weak stomach or are eating while reading this, you might want to put the book down. You've been warned.

Anyway, the colon is at the base of your intestines and is the last place where food ends up before it's eliminated from the body. Now, any animal—such as a lion, vulture, or hyena—that's designed by nature to eat meat needs to get the decaying, putrefying flesh out of its body as quickly as possible. So it should come as no surprise that these meat-eaters don't have colons to slow down the process. To further expedite things, these animals possess hydrochloric acids in their stomachs that are twenty times stronger than our digestive acids. On top of all that, carnivorous animals have a small intestine that's only three to six times the length of their body. Ours is ten times the length of the human body. Still think you were put on earth to eat defenseless animals?

So what happens to a hot dog (which, by the way, is made from ground-up animal lips, assholes, and other nasty by-products that are injected into a condom-like casing made out of intestines) as it makes its way out of your body? Well, meat doesn't contain any fiber, which means that it doesn't pass through our digestive tract easily. So while it sits there in our intestines waiting for the next step, some of the rotting flesh is absorbed into the bloodstream through the intestinal walls. This toxic shit is then spread throughout your body, increasing your risk for heart disease, stroke, cancer, high blood pressure, and many other diseases. And even after the majority of digested meat makes its way out of your body, a percentage of it remains behind, just putrefying in your intestines and colon. I personally know a colonic irrigation specialist (aka professional enema practitioner), and the ancient shit he's seen coming out of people's asses could be material for a horror flick. Meat-eaters have nasty colons. Listen, I know everybody's shit stinks, but one day I let this overweight, meat-eating dude who worked on my apartment use my bathroom. The stench from that dump hung around for a week. Literally. Turns out he had eaten pig knuckles and chitlins for dinner the night before. Well, I learned my lesson, and now I have a sign hanging above my toilet that reads VEGETARIANS ONLY. And, no, I'm not shitting you.

END THE VICIOUS CYCLE

The further away we get from organic, whole, plant-based foods, the more health problems we face. So how do we get off this roller coaster and make the necessary changes? The first thing you need to do is cut back on your meat consumption. You'd be surprised by how easy it is to replace that disgusting, poisonous meat with delicious combinations of fruits, veggies, whole grains, beans, nuts, seeds, and endless other options. Next on the list is eliminating processed foods from your diet—you especially want to stay away from anything containing artificial colors, flavors, hydrogenated oils, preservatives, added sugars, and artificial sweeteners. And then there's exercise: even if you're out of shape, set aside some time for a little light exercise each day. Walking, stretching, or doing some basic yoga is a great, simple way to start. You've gotta get your blood to flow like a raging river instead of a stagnant pond. When the blood's flowing, the body works to get rid of toxins.

A healthy life is a marathon, not a sprint, so pace yourself with little changes in your daily lifestyle and you'll see amazing results. Once you stop eating the bad stuff, you may notice some pussies acne or other minor skin ailments. Don't be alarmed. That's a sign that your body is detoxing. Toxins are eliminated through the skin, and as your health progresses it will clear up. As your body eliminates toxins, you'll also notice increased bowel movements. Forget about taking laxatives or enemas; this is the natural way to get rid of that rancid shit. When I was working on an album with my band, we recorded up in Rhode Island at a place called Normandy Sound. The owner of the studio, Phil, was overweight and he ate the worst shit all day long. Well, one morning he forgot to lock the bathroom door and I walked in on him injecting his Fleet enema up his asshole, because he couldn't take a dump unless he used it. After that we called him the Admiral of the Fleet. I'm still in therapy from the sight of it. Poor Phil is an extreme example, but a lot of people use laxatives, enemas, and fiber pills to get them going—and they think that's normal. The truth is, you should never need any of that crap. As long as you eat properly to maintain healthy colon function, your body will figure out the rest. When I hear dudes grunting in the gym bathroom like they're benching three hundred pounds, something ain't right.

If you're detoxing off shitty foods and need a little help to get things moving, here's a shortcut: get a colonic (aka colon hydrotherapy). It's a treatment that washes out all the sick shit that's built up in your colon. A friend of mine who is a colonic therapist broke it down for me. He said that colonics "create an environment where the organs can purge toxins from the various tissues with innate healing wisdom. The body then circulates toxins into the passages of elimination, and colonics assist the body in completely removing the toxins as quickly as possible." He went on to add that removing stored toxins allows "the body to breathe again, rejuvenates the tissues, and restores a balanced and harmonious chemistry." Colonics aren't a new diet or program; they're part of a healthy lifestyle that gives you vibrancy and vitality. My boy Ishmael delivers colonics and has shown me photos of the crazy stuff that came out of the many people he has helped. In fact, parasites from different types of undercooked meat can fester undetected in the intestines and cause serious health problems down the road. He also showed me how people's health improved as they changed their diets and got regular colonics. In one case, he had several pictures of a guy who had the worst case of psoriasis I'd ever seen. As he followed Ishmael's dietary advice and got colonics, his body healed until the psoriasis was entirely gone.

I strongly believe, as does Ishmael, that you can quickly eliminate all that poisonous fecal matter you got from eating meat through colonics. I can't stress enough how important proper colon care is. If your bowel movements are becoming less frequent, you need to take this information very seriously. If you're eating and nothing's coming out, all of that diseased fecal matter has to be sitting somewhere—and now you know where.

So laugh if you want, tough guy, but your colon is where disease starts. You ever see old people who had to get a colostomy? They shit into a sack through their abdomen and carry around a bag of their own feces everywhere they go. I beg you to stick your nose in there and take a whiff; you'd never lay your eyes on meat again. But remember: we didn't get this way overnight, and the goal here is gradual improvement. Don't try to go hard-core and think, "That's it! I'm doing seven colonics a week and eating nothing but alfalfa sprouts!" Your body cannot handle such a dramatic change of pace—and that is a very bad way to detox. Trust me.

THE HEALING POWER OF GREEN FOODS

Throughout my years of using natural foods as medicines, I can genuinely vouch for their amazing healing powers. But it's important to remember that we have to stop eating the bad stuff to see the benefits of the good stuff. Just recently I told someone suffering from joint problems about the amazing healing properties of MSM, or methylsulfonylmethane (organic sulfurs from the ocean). He said he tried it and it didn't work for him. And then one day I noticed him eating a huge piece of red meat. When I told him to cut back on meat and other acid-producing foods (like potatoes, peppers, raw tomatoes, and eggplant), he said, point blank, "No way, guy." So there you have it; don't expect to see the benefits of whole foods if you're canceling out your own efforts with shitty foods.

The idea here is to help your body to heal itself, and for that to happen you need to keep your immune system fired up. One way to do that, as we've already discussed, is to keep your pH level in the alkaline range. (Turn to pages 18–19 for a list of alkaline foods.) Another easy way to reduce the acid in your blood is to incorporate wheatgrass juice into your diet. Wheatgrass has an abundance of alkaline minerals, and not only reduces overacidity in the blood, but has a bunch of other benefits: it's been proven to stimulate the metabolism and successfully treat ulcers, constipation, diarrhea, and other issues involving the gastrointestinal tract. Wheatgrass is also full of amino acids (seventeen of them), which are crucial for cell renewal, not to mention valuable vitamins, minerals, chlorophyll, and enzymes.

Chlorella, a type of green algae the Japanese have been incorporating into their diet for centuries, is another amazing example of a detoxifying plant. Chlorella contains all eight essential amino acids and more than twenty vitamins and minerals. Better yet, it naturally filters out dangerous toxins (alcohol, pesticides, heavy metals like mercury, etc.) from your body. And if that isn't enough, it also helps to strengthen your immune system, digest your food, and freshen your breath.

Clearly green foods can heal us. I learned about the nutritional power of algae from an Ironman triathlete friend of mine. Chlorella, spirulina, and AFA (aphanizomenon flos-aquae) are algae that increase your energy and stamina and boost your immune system. From my own personal experience, I can attest to their strengthening power and healing benefits. Chlorella is even used to prevent and fight cancer, reduce the effects of radiation, and boost the production of white blood cells.[28]

Wheatgrass and algae are also loaded with iron, which is something anyone following a plant-based diet needs to monitor closely, since most people rely on red meat for their iron needs. Women lose iron during menstruation and are especially at risk for anemia, but the fellas also gotta make sure this new diet has enough iron to maintain their health. Sometimes doctors may recommend iron supplements, but this inorganic iron isn't always absorbed properly by your body and can cause constipation. A simple glass of citrus juice with two tablespoons of blackstrap molasses is a great, natural iron booster. Or try a nice dose of spinach, which is packed with iron. You can even cook your food in a cast-iron pan and some of the mineral will leach into your food (this is a good thing).

A POUND OF PREVENTION = A TON OF CURES

We need to reverse the terrible damage we've done to our bodies. We're directly responsible for some of this damage—including the bad food, prescription and recreational drugs, alcohol, and cigarettes—but there's a lot that we're not in control of. Half of our food crops are genetically modified Frankencrops that get sprayed with a ton of pesticides, which are toxic for the environment and our bodies (turn to the Appendix, page 257, for details on this). Pollution from giant livestock farms is a real threat to our health, too, since thousands of animals together produce an unreal amount of manure.[29] And animals kept in filthy, inhumane feedlots are treated with growth hormones and steroids[30] and antibiotics[31] to ward off diseases (though the USDA will sometimes make a carcass passable for inspection by simply cutting off the diseased body parts),[32] and all of those drugs may or may not make their way into your dinner, too.

And, by the way, the raw meat you see at the superstore has been treated with sodium nitrite to slow down decay and give it that bright red color (untreated meat has a gray, sickly look). This doesn't seem so bad, right? Wrong. Recent studies have shown there may be a link between sodium nitrites and colon cancer.[33] Now, get ready to have your fuckin' world rocked. Every time you enjoy a glass of wine or a pint of beer with your meat dinner, you're creating a deadly chemical reaction in your stomach. As chemicals in the wine and beer react with nitrites in the meat, dangerous chemical compounds called nitrosamines are formed. When meat treated with nitrites or nitrates is cooked at high temperatures, that also creates nitrosamines. Here's how dangerous they are: they are a known carcinogen![34]

The point is, we are being poisoned every day by the meat and poultry industries, and we are willingly ingesting their poison; but if we take preventative measures to stay healthy, we'll be amazed at how the immune system can fight off disease. The knowledge is out there, but it's up to us to make the change and allow our bodies to detox and heal. I've been all over the world in my travels, and I find that we Americans are greatly lagging behind in dietary knowledge. We may have thousands of weapons to fight off enemies, but we are killing ourselves with what we eat.

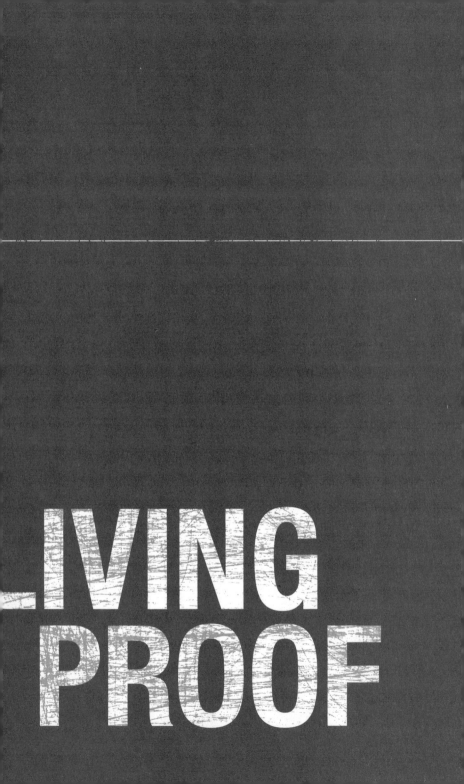

LIVING PROOF

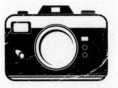

Just so we're clear on the whole "lacking protein" thing . . . All these dudes are plant-based ass-kickers!

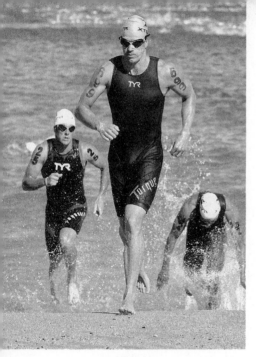

RIP ESSELSTYN

AUTHOR, *THE ENGINE 2 DIET*,
FIREFIGHTER, TRIATHLETE, AND
STUD MOTHER-EFFER.

JAKE SHIELDS

BADASS, MIXED MARTIAL
ARTS CHAMPION.

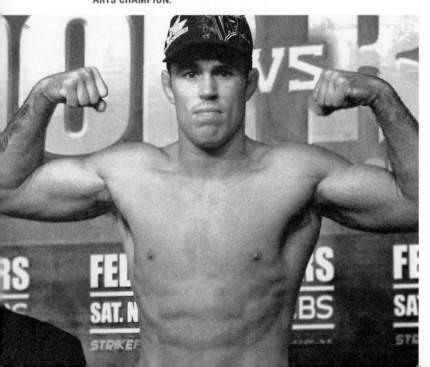

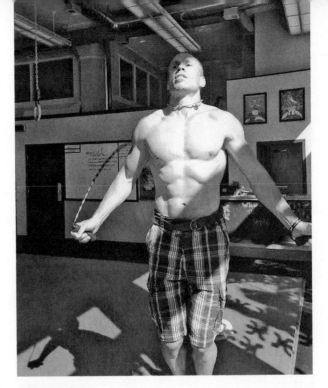

JON HINDS

BRAZILIAN JIUJITSU BLACK BELT GOLD MEDALIST (PAN AM GAMES)

FOUNDER OF MONKEY BAR GYM . . . BEAST!!!

FRED BISCI

A SPECIAL SHOUT OUT TO MY MAN, FRED. HE IS EIGHTY-FOUR
YEARS YOUNG, HAS BEEN PLANT-BASED FOR SIXTY YEARS,
AND STILL RUNS TEN MILES A DAY!

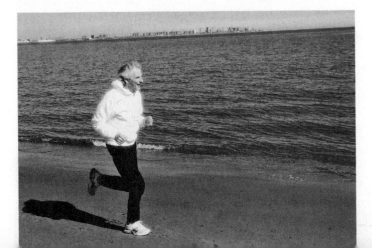

MIKE MAHLER

AUTHOR, *LIVE LIFE AGGRESSIVELY*,
KETTLEBELL INSTRUCTOR, AND A
FRIGGIN' BEAST!

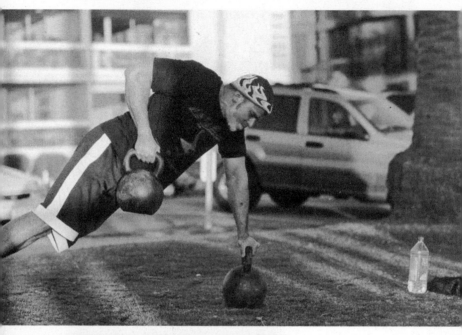

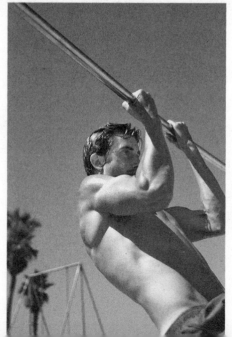

BRENDAN BRAZIER

AUTHOR, *THE THRIVE DIET*,
IRONMAN, AND TWO-TIME
CANADIAN 50K ULTRA-
MARATHON CHAMP.

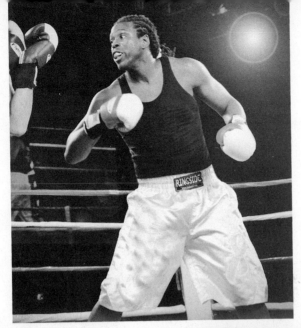

CAM AWESOME

PROFESSOR OF THE
SWEET SCIENCE.

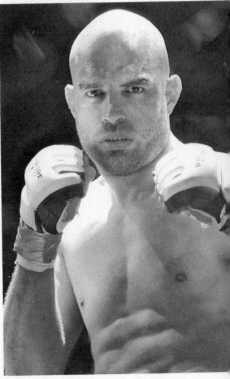

JAMES "LIGHTNING" WILKS

UFC ULTIMATE FIGHTER CHAMPION,
FOUNDER, LIGHTNING MMA.

(DEREK HAMILTON)

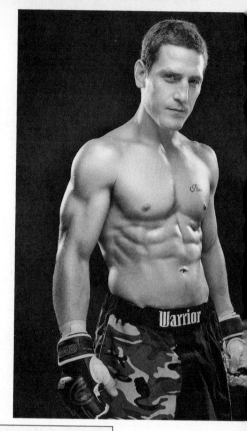

MAC DANZIG

**UFC ULTIMATE FIGHTER
CHAMPION.**

(MELISSA SCHWARTZ/SCHWARTZ
STUDIOS)

RICH ROLL

**ULTRA-IRONMAN AND
AUTHOR, *FINDING ULTRA*,
VOTED ONE OF THE WORLD'S
TOP 25 FITTEST MEN.**

(JOHN SEGESTA)

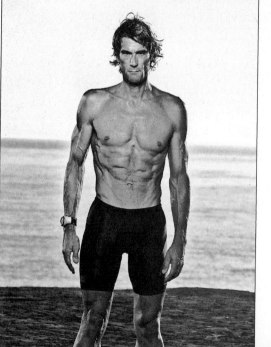

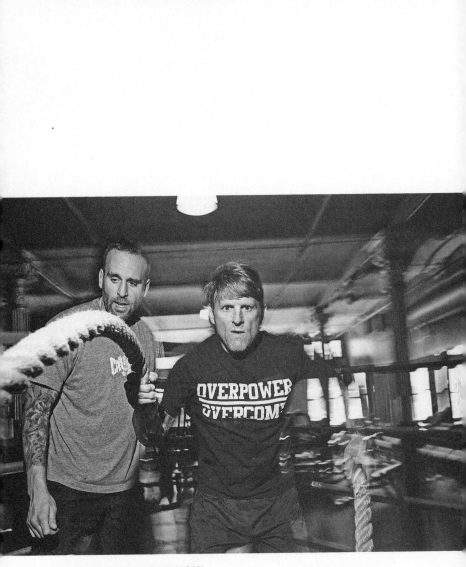

AARON DROGOSZEWSKI

ME, TRAINING FOR AN IRONMAN, WITH BADASS
TRAINER AARON DROGOSZEWSKI.

(RAY LEGO)

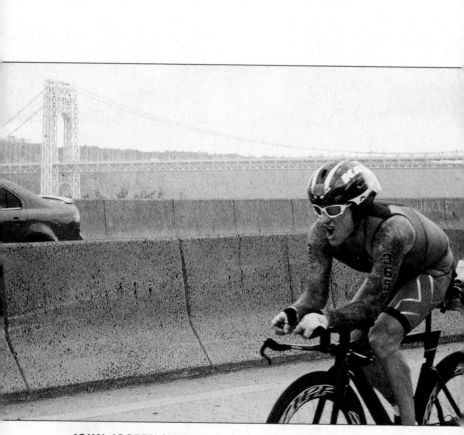

JOHN JOSEPH (ME)

COMPETING IN THE NYC TRIATHLON.

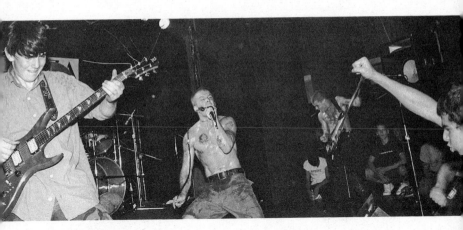

JOHN JOSEPH

YOURS TRULY, AGE TWENTY-TWO IN 1984 (TOP).
STILL ROCKIN' HARD TWENTY-FIVE YEARS LATER (BOTTOM).

(JOSEPH HENDERSON)

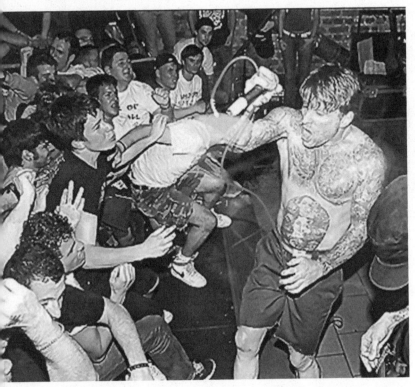

CHAPTER 8

THE BULLSHIT PROTEIN MYTH

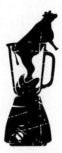

THE BULLSHIT PROTEIN MYTH

Meatheads Are So 1980

Why is it when I mention to some wannabe macho men that I eat a 100 percent plant-based diet, their immediate reaction is to go on the attack, defending *their* way of eating? They get pissed-off and combative, unleashing a torrent of unproven verbal diarrhea. "What are you talking about, man, that's retarded, humans are designed to eat meat. You don't get enough vitamins." Well, given that vitamins come from plants, I get more vitamins by breakfast than you eat in a week. Anything else? Oh yeah, then there's this genius insight: "If we didn't eat animals they would overpopulate the planet." Fact: we breed animals for slaughter and for that reason farm animals outnumber human beings by a 65:1 ratio in the United States. It's not like we're chasing them down in the wild like our ancestors had to do, when it was either eat or be eaten. Nature managed to thin the herds just fine before the slaughterhouse scumbags started their factory farm operations.

One of these meatheads even went on a Facebook rant for several days trying to defeat me, only to admit on the third day that he was sixty pounds overweight and had undergone bypass surgery at the age of thirty-seven. So, let me get this straight: eating an organic, plant-based diet is not natural, but cracking your chest open like a friggin' walnut, taking a vein out of your leg, and sewing it into your coronary artery is?

And of course no discussion on the subject would be complete without the number-one, redundant, unproven, idiot question of all time: "Meat is man-food. If you don't eat it, where the hell you gonna get your protein, dude?"

So now I feel I must take it upon myself to smash, obliterate, and choke the fuck out of a false accusation that meat-eaters so often throw at us plant-eaters: the Bullshit Protein Myth.

Sometimes the fact that I've been plant-based for about thirty-three years comes up at the gym. These dudes look at me—I'm a solid guy at five foot nine and 170 pounds—and assume there's no way I could be a veggie. Some of them have heard that not eating meat can be good for you, but they worry about getting skinny and weak like a lot of the vegetarians and vegans they see. Before getting deep into a biology lesson with our Neanderthal friends, I try to relate to them on their prehistoric level. "You're pretty strong, bro . . . what do you bench? Around two fifty? Yeah? Impressive, but stay with me on this: Are you stronger than a bull, rhino, elephant, horse, or gorilla? No? Well, every one of those creatures is a vegetarian." After I rope these fools in, I explain that they can get their protein from great plant-based sources that won't damage their kidneys or other essential organs, or send their cholesterol through the roof.

I tell them that foods like tofu (soybean curd), seitan (a delicious wheat-based meat substitute), tempeh (soybeans in cake form), quinoa (a whole grain that is also a complete protein source), veggie burgers, and some good old rice and beans are delicious examples of protein-rich foods that are plant based. We've already discussed the detoxifying properties of chlorella, a type of green algae. Well, chlorella is also loaded with something called albumin, an essential protein that's abundant in healthy people and low in critically sick people. Lecithin is another amazing plant-based protein supplement, and it has been proven to significantly lower your cholesterol. It blows these guys away when I tell them they can make a superfood shake with these ingredients (you'll find the recipe for it on page 187) that contains more than 30 grams of protein—good enough for any workout or recovery. In the past, I've had nothing but one of these shakes and gone on a seventy-mile bike ride with some sick-ass climbs. Try accomplishing that after eating a quarter-pounder with cheese.

Nowadays I answer these dumb questions by asking intelligent ones. "Bro, where do you get your chlorophyll, vitamin K, flavonoids, phytonutrients, selenium, live-food enzymes, or beta-carotene?" You see the point I'm making here? Why have we been programmed to think that protein is the *only thing we need* for power and it can *only be found* in the flesh and organ meats of an animal, so if I'm not consuming putrid, rotting, decaying corpses then I couldn't possibly be getting enough protein?

Little by little, the truth about animal protein is getting out. The USDA has already readjusted the food pyramid—that big lie I was force-fed as a kid—to suggest we get more protein, and even cereal boxes are telling you to eat more fiber. After I explain all this to the gym rats I encounter, the next thing they say is, "So what do you eat . . . salads?" I laugh when I hear that, and I ask them, "What did you eat last night? Or the night before? Or the night before that?" Usually they eat the same boring, poisonous foods dinner after dinner. I'm a damn good cook who specializes in a variety of healthy, great-tasting, and nutrient-rich meals. Anytime I have a staunch meat-eater over for dinner

I hear the same thing: "Man, you fooled me. I didn't even miss the meat."

Don't believe the hype about meat and protein. You need only about 56 grams of protein a day, which is roughly the amount in a cup each of beans and brown rice and a peanut butter sandwich on whole wheat bread.[35] I implore you to question your assumptions about how much protein you need. There are so many more factors in keeping the body healthy and strong than just protein consumption. Everyone seems to think that working out and adding muscle means ingesting jugs of protein. But too much protein will make you fat, just like anything else. Sure, we need protein to rebuild and repair muscle, but that protein doesn't need to come from animals. So now for the benefit of all the rocket scientists out there who tried to give me a lecture, let's take a look at how our bodies actually convert the food we eat into the energy that keeps us alive, and what role protein plays in that process.

CONVERTING FOOD INTO POWER

Digestion begins as the enzymes in your saliva start to break down food as you chew it. After you swallow it, the food then travels to the stomach via the esophagus. There digestion continues for another two to six hours, depending upon the type of food you ate. This process reduces food into molecules that the body can then use for producing energy. Most nutrient absorption occurs in the small intestine, while water absorption occurs in the large intestine.

Your body relies primarily on carbohydrates and fats from the foods you eat for energy. The blood transports these chemicals to the cells of your body through your veins and arteries (aka your circulatory system). Within your cells are little fuel-processing plants called mitochondria. This is where energy production occurs through a complex series of chemical reactions to produce something called ATP (adenosine triphosphate), which is the energy currency in your body. The circulatory system also transports oxygen from the lungs to cells throughout your body so that this process, known as cellular respiration, can take place.

Now, if you start that whole process off by putting toxins in your body, that is, meat, eggs, fish, dairy, and heavily processed foods—all of which are acid forming and in some cases take days to digest—you are creating a backup in the small intestine and preventing the rest of the energy-producing process from operating efficiently.

In his amazing book, *Your Healthy Journey*, Fred Bisci

talks about "food sequencing" for optimum health and vitality. In other words you should "stack" what you are eating throughout the day in this order: water, raw juice, raw foods, and then cooked food. Why? Because if you place raw foods or juice on top of cooked foods like grains, beans, etc., which take four to six hours to digest, they will ferment and thus you will lose their nutritional benefits. Raw foods, especially fresh-pressed juice, become assimilated almost immediately because they have their own live enzymes to help in absorption and digestion. So when you sequence what you eat you get all the power from these foods. Nothing is wasted.

Bisci also says that meat contains dangerous nitrogen gas, which does a number on your immune system. "Your body recognizes that it doesn't want the over-stimulation of the nitrogenous by-products, the ammonia and the urea. Ammonia is not supposed to stay in your body very long at all. It's converted to urea. Then you try to get rid of urea when you urinate. Uric acid, urea, all these types of things, do not belong in your system."

All of that uric acid and urea—the by-products from the breakdown of ammonia—can lead to gout. You will never see a person who eats a clean plant-based or raw-food diet have gout. It is the result of your body processing animal protein.

The funny thing is that women rarely continue to argue

the point of eating animal protein once they hear all of this science explained properly. It's the men who go on and on, stuck on stupid, thinking that not eating meat will make them less manly, that they need animal protein—and lots of it—to be strong. So they consume either tons of chicken, steak, and eggs, or gallons of preservative-filled protein powders. Guys, if you do use a protein enhancer, you have to get with the program. Stop buying those three-gallon jugs at GNC with some Neanderthal, steroided-out bodybuilder on the label. There are so many organic, clean, plant-based protein supplement products. I use different organic varieties when I travel that are loaded with plant-based superfoods and more than an ample amount of protein. And when I do make a smoothie or protein shake, I always add fresh organic greens like spinach to offset the acidity of the protein.

Another thing these guys tend to overlook is the fact that performance isn't just about how much power you have; it's about how long you can exude that power. In other words: endurance. The military test for fitness covers three areas: flexibility, strength, and endurance. Without endurance, the other two don't matter—you're just a dude who can do a split and bench 250. I mean, ladies you agree, right? I'm sure you've had your share of two-pump chumps. No fun, is it? Guys, if you want real endurance and power, meat ain't gonna cut it.

As a matter of fact, some of the world's top athletes are vegetarians: six-time Ironman triathlon winner Dave Scott, Heisman Trophy winner Desmond Howard, UFC lightweight fighter Mac Danzig, middleweight boxing champ Keith Holmes, Ironman Brendan Brazier, Olympic 400-meter hurdles gold medalist Edwin Moses, Olympic wrestling medal winner Chris Campbell, EPIC5 finisher Rich Roll, fitness guru Mike Mahler, world-class body-builder Bill Pearl, natural bodybuilding champion Robert Cheeke, MMA fighter Jake Shields, Olympic sprinter Carl Lewis . . . the list of stud motherfuckers who realized meat is for pussies goes on and on. By eating smaller, well-balanced, plant-based meals throughout the day, you can keep your endurance level up and your metabolism burning fat all day long.

People who eat a meat-based diet often consume twice as much protein as they need—and excess protein is no good for your body. In fact, it can contribute to osteoporosis and kidney stones, since animal protein raises the acid level in our blood, causing calcium to be excreted from the bones to restore the blood's natural pH balance. The excreted calcium ends up in the kidneys, where it can form kidney stones or even trigger kidney disease.

People write to me all the time and most tell me that after just a couple of weeks of going meat-free they feel great and have more energy. That's because they're not impacting their colons with putrefying flesh. Some people who were eating a lot of animal protein and had a very high toxicity in their bodies feel weak and tired at first and immediately assume it's because they're not getting enough protein. I can assure you that as long as you eat plenty of clean, plant-based protein and continue on, all of that will pass and you will get stronger than ever before.

Hopefully even the most die-hard meathead readers are now coming around to the idea that you don't need to eat a cow to be as strong as a bull. And if not, let me drop some wisdom here from my Ironman friend Brendan Brazier, who also happens to formulate a line of plant-based products for athletes.

ME: How does protein consumption impact athletic performance? What should we eat to fuel our workouts?

BRENDAN: Well, protein is more for rebuilding and repairing and complex carbohydrates are more for fueling. You have to make sure you don't consume too much protein prior to training because your body has to convert that to usable fuel. Now, it can do that, but it's not as efficient, it's not as clean as using carbs for energy. So what happens is then there's a chemical reaction, and if you've ever smelled people in the gym giving off that ammonia smell, that's actually a result of consuming too much protein before their workout and their body has to make that conversion. So ideally you want to eat complex carbohydrates to fuel your workouts and a clean, plant-based protein after to rebuild and repair.

ME: So what are the best sources of protein?

BRENDAN: The best protein sources are the ones that also have a high mineral content because minerals are alkaline forming and protein is acid forming. So you want to make sure when you have protein you get it with minerals so it offsets the acidity. That's going to help reduce inflammation. Also anything containing chlorophyll, anything green, any kind of green protein. Hemp is a great source. Even things like spinach, kale, seaweed, and the algaes are amazing, too; they contain anywhere from forty-five percent to sixty-five percent protein. A lot of people don't really realize how high greens are in protein and they're exceptional to use because they contain chlorophyll, which will help reduce inflammation yet still allow the body to rebuild and repair after exercise, which is essential because if you aren't inflamed you don't have to move the muscles as much. If you look at any endurance athlete, say for instance all the muscle contractions needed by anyone doing triathlons or marathons, well, if you have to work harder for every muscle contraction that will definitely impede your performance. Why would you want to spend more energy than you need to? So getting that quality green, mineral-rich protein right after a workout is going to help a lot.

DIETS ARE FOR JERK-OFFS

CHAPTER 9

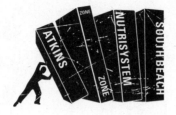

DIETS ARE FOR JERK-OFFS

By now I think I've presented you with enough evidence to establish that we have become a nation of sick, miserable, morbidly obese pussies. And just like the food manufacturers, the pharmaceutical companies, and slick advertising firms that have profited by leading us down the road to becoming fat-asses, there's another industry waiting to profit from your feeble attempts to shed the weight you never should have gained in the first place: the weight loss industry. These fuckers are up there with Big Pharma in terms of profits—with 100 million dieters it's a $20 billion-a-year industry, promising America with celebrity endorsements and magic formulas that we can get skinny if we buy their products and follow their advice.

But the solution to our health crisis isn't a diet. Diets are for jerk-offs. They address only one part of the problem—being fat—not necessarily being *healthy*. They also don't work in the long term—that's why they're called "diets." If they worked long term, no one would ever need to "diet" again.

Here's a word no dieting pussy ever wants to hear: *balance*. Every dieter I know takes their cues from the latest fad diet, spending days, weeks, months, and sometimes even years eating shitty food and abusing their bodies. Dieters don't care about the nutrition they're putting in their bodies—the fuel they're feeding their cells; they care about calories. Well, fuck, you can eat 100 calories of bacon lard and french fries, and you might be skinny, but the inside of your body is still going to look like shit.

Let me tell you about a guy I know. He eats shit, gets drunk night after night, smokes cigarettes, doesn't exercise, and is under constant stress, but then he goes on his AMAZING 21-Day "Miracle Cleanse Diet" where he only drinks a combination of lemon juice, cayenne, and maple syrup for every meal to supposedly "detox" his body. By day ten I'm ready to call the psych ward to have that fucker carted off in a straitjacket.

All of your weight issues stemming from not wanting to control your taste buds and overcome laziness need to end now. Today. No bullshit. Even if you have a bad case of Dunlap disease (your belly dun lapped over your belt), you've gotta accept the fact that diets don't work. They are for weak-minded people who want the magic bullet.

I don't diet. I make proper food choices every day. If I decide to eat some fried veggie food a couple of days a week . . . big fuckin' deal! You can't approach food with too rigid of an attitude. Here's my philosophy: It's better to let someone eat a little processed vegetarian food or fake meat in the beginning than to have them go back to eating a poisonous meat diet. If they keep at it they will eventually transition out of it for the most part. I did. I still have an occasional piece of seitan, but that's my thing. Everyone has their thing. The point is, food is one of the great pleasures in life and any diet or too-strict food regimen takes all the joy out of that. You've gotta let your balls breathe a little or you're gonna crash and burn. Moderation and balance are key to having fun in life.

This diet shit has gotten out of hand over the past decade, hasn't it? We made Jared, the nerdy Subway sandwich guy, into a household name for eating processed meat, cheese, and bread that was low in calories. If these diets are so great, why are we still the fattest fuckin' nation on earth? The truth is that yo-yo dieting and crash courses on health only make you sicker. All of these options focus on the short term; then, when you gain the weight back, those diet fuckers throw you the next sensation. You look everywhere for the answers and never find them. Don't make your life—and more important, your happiness—more difficult than it needs to be.

Going plant-based will require you to monitor all of what you're ingesting daily. That means reading labels if you do buy anything packaged, which, believe it or not, you will eventually stop doing for the most part except for a few specialty items. When you enter a supermarket you'll pass right by those aisles of processed food as well as the morgue (meat section) and find your way to the whole-food and organic produce sections. And have you ever paid attention to how food is placed in supermarkets? Do you think it's laid out that way by chance? Hell no it isn't: it's strategic. They actually have people with college degrees in marketing figuring that shit out. They want you to have to travel like a mouse in a maze, making your way through their aisles of poison before you get to the fruit and vegetable section, and they hope your tongue will drag you down along the way.

Don't let it. Remember the Stop and Think Mechanism. Remember to pause and use your intelligence over the impulses of your senses. That's the way to avoid the pitfalls not only in the supermarket, but in the face of the crap being thrown at you on a daily basis by these marketing fuckers on TV pushing the latest diet fad on you.

THE SHIT LIST

So let's get down to business, shall we? The following are my thoughts on some of the most bullshit diets out there.

SOUTH BEACH DIET

My biggest problem with this one is that it doesn't stress exercise enough. The plan suggests that twenty minutes each day will do. Bullshit. That's fine if you're already in shape, but everyone's body type is different, and overweight people need much more exercise than that. If you're spending forty minutes eating and only twenty exercising, I don't like your chances for losing weight. Also, the diet doesn't take allergies into consideration, and a lot of people need to avoid some of the mainstays of that diet (dairy, eggs, etc.). And come on, commercial pasteurized dairy? There are growth hormones, pesticides, and bacteria in there, bros! South Beach recommends eating a lot of fish, too—fish that's often loaded with contaminants and mercury. It also encourages the use of aspartame, the artificial sweetener commonly marketed as NutraSweet or Equal. That shit is pure chemicals and actually increases sugar cravings. Don't buy it.

ZONE DIET

Any diet that makes it this black-and-white—40 percent of your calories from carbs, 30 percent from fat, and 30 percent from protein—is bullshit. The Zone diet stresses lean meat, egg whites, poultry, and fish—industries that are poisonous for you and your planet—but lacks fruits, veggies, fiber, and complex carbs. When are these fuckers gonna man up and look at our physiological makeup? We have a colon, you fuckin' idiots. Also, any diet this structured is eventually going to drive you bananas. When you do go off it (which most people do because of its rigidity and the fact that its cost may compel you to take out a second mortgage), the little weight you've lost is quickly regained. So is it really worth the inevitable health risks? These douche bags need to stop shitting on complex carbs; they were around for tens of thousands of years before these scumbags found a way to cheat you with idiotic systems of weight loss.

ATKINS DIET

Not as many people are swearing by the Atkins bullshit nowadays, but the namesake doctor scammed hordes of people with Atkins-branded products on every shelf before he kicked the bucket. At the peak of this meat-heavy trend, he had people so brainwashed that the grain producers were undergoing the worst times in recent memory. Dr. Atkins may have died in 2003 from slipping on ice, but the truth is that he had a history of heart problems. So it should come as no surprise that his wife, who stood to lose millions, tried to block the coroner's report that outlined how Dr. Atkins's problems arose from years of practicing what he preached.

NUTRISYSTEM

Ever wonder why this shit doesn't need to be refrigerated? Because it's processed fuckin' garbage loaded with preservatives! This diet fails because anyone who has been on it would agree that the food—and I use the term loosely—tastes like shit. But man oh man, those turd meals look good on TV. They must have called in Steven Spielberg for some special effects. Cakes, cookies, hot dogs, hamburgers, mac and cheese . . . motherfucker, please! This is nothing but junk food disguised as healthy eating, so don't give these chumps a dime. Can't you control your own portion sizes and tell them to fuck off? Bro, do yourself a favor and save the three hundred dollars each month.

SPRINKLE DIET

Dig this . . . you sprinkle this poisonous processed shit called "Sensa" on your food and it makes everything you eat saltier or sweeter and supposedly tricks you into thinking you're full. Well, first off, overweight people who are eating themselves to an early death still eat even when they are full, and who cares if the FDA gave their approval? And what exactly is in Sensa? Pay attention because the devil is always in the details. Maltodextrin (highly processed from GMO corn or potatoes); natural and artificial flavors (uh, you probably mean MSG, don't you?), FD&C Yellow, Carmine (made from dried ground-up beetles); soy and milk ingredients (GMO soy and milk loaded with hormones). *Pass!*

I don't care what your sister or your girlfriend or your buddy at the gym says; you've gotta recognize diets for what they are: a way for a pussy to take a shortcut instead of doing real work. There are no shortcuts to health and sustainable weight loss. If you want to lose weight, then eat smart, prepare balanced plant-based meals, and exercise. It takes commitment, it takes patience, it takes determination. But if you're willing to do that, you've got a real shot at squeezing into that Speedo this summer. Actually . . . spare us the sight.

SOME LIKE IT RAW

Eating mainly organic, raw foods is a great way to lose weight, stay healthy, and kick your libido into the fucking stratosphere. Uncooked and unprocessed vegetables, fruits, nuts, and seeds contain live enzymes and are super-healthy and easy to digest. Naturally, if your body uses less energy to digest these foods than it does to digest heavy meat, fish, egg, dairy, and even vegetarian greaseball meals, you'll feel lighter and more energetic. I never feel bloated after a raw meal.

Personally, I find it hard to be 100 percent raw living in New York City in the winter. I like my hot organic oatmeal and soups. Most of the completely raw food peeps I know made a beeline for warmer climates. Since most of us don't have that luxury, let's be realistic. I highly encourage incorporating raw foods into your diet, as they help to eliminate all that vile, impacted crap sitting in your swollen colon. Don't be alarmed if you experience increased bowel movements at first; it just means your body is healing itself. And if you've got the kind of gas that could send the hotties running for the hills, no big deal. Just chew better, try to eat your raw foods early in the day, and go pick up some Beano.

The classic example of the power of raw foods is a woman named Angela Stokes. She was in the news a few years back for losing 160 pounds over a span of two years. "My mobility was quite restricted . . . I was unwilling to participate in things from cutting my toenails to going on a walk with my friends," remembered Angela. "I tried to give this impression that I felt fine about everything, but inside I was in a lot of pain a lot of the time."

While Angela was working at a greenhouse in Iceland, her friend lent her a copy of a book about the health benefits of eating raw foods. She stopped eating meat, animal products, and processed foods and started eating raw that very next day. "Everything in my life completely shifted. It was like a lightbulb moment to be like . . . 'this is what I was waiting for to reclaim my health.'

"To me, the thing with raw food is that it just makes sense. It's simple and natural, eating food straight from the earth. There's no rocket science, no mystery," said Angela. "Once you understand the simple principle that no other animal in the wild eats cooked or processed foods, that's it." Thanks to eating raw foods, Angela's emotional, physical, and social well-being have never been better.

Fellas, take this chick's lead; put that fucking doughnut down, and get with the program. And I know there are a few of you guys out there who haven't seen places on your bodies in quite some time, too. So clean up your act with some raw food, get a colonic, and get your bowels and asses moving.

SIX-PACK OR KEG? YOUR CHOICE

Between living in New York City and traveling around the world, I've heard more than enough foreigners talk about how shocked they are by the portion sizes we eat in America. Just the other day, an Englishman told me he gained fifteen pounds in the one week he spent in the States. Here's the point: fixing your diet isn't just about changing *what* you eat, but how *much of it* you put into your body. That's why I eat four to five smaller, nutrient-dense, plant-based meals throughout the day. Smaller meals are like high-octane fuel for the body; they keep your engines burning on all cylinders. On the other hand, people who skip meals tend to overeat when they finally sit down.[36] Worse yet, when you don't eat for a long period of time your metabolism slows down to conserve energy.

The only way you'll actually lose weight and reduce fat levels around your midsection is by burning off more calories than you're taking in and developing a solid exercise plan. I love to do a forty-five-minute mix of cardio and abdominals; it's a beast for getting toned. (You'll get plenty more exercise and meal plan pointers in chapters 12 and 13.)

Truth be told, there is no healthy way to get immediate, drastic weight loss, let alone a six-pack—and diets are definitely not the answer. But if you devote yourself to making small changes every day, like keeping your portion sizes in check and working out, the benefits will come. You'll feel better, look better, and even have a positive mental attitude (PMA). Chicks pick up on that, and let's get real, you probably went on a diet in the first place to impress the ladies. But don't be a jerk-off pussy dieter who gains the weight back. That failure will make you feel like shit. With a natural, plant-based approach, you're guaranteed a lifetime of looking like a stud on the inside and the outside.

MEAT AND YOUR MEAT

We all know that sex sells. So if I can't convince your big head to rethink your eating and exercise habits, maybe appealing to your little head will be a fuckin' wake-up call.

As you know by now, eating meat puts you at risk for terrifying health issues like heart disease, diabetes, and cancer, which could change your life forever. But avoiding meat, and the toxic chemicals it contains, helps keep you disease-free.

Now what does all of this have to do with the health of your junk, you ask? Well, when you eat a bunch of animal products, you're also more likely to have high cholesterol. Cholesterol is a plaquelike substance that has a tendency to build up in your arteries and veins and restrict blood flow to important organs—like your heart. In an ideal world, your blood courses through your veins like a white-water rapid. So, fellas, shouldn't you be worried that cholesterol from the meat you're consuming like a caveman is also blocking the flow of blood to your main vein?

An estimated 20 to 30 million men suffer from erectile dysfunction (ED).[37] Now, when your compass stops pointing north, it means the blood's not flowing like it did in the good old days. But you don't need drugs like Viagra, Cialis, or whatever else; that shit's for pussies. Let's say you're going to Jamaica with your hot new girlfriend and the moron at Homeland Security loses your pills. Chances are she's gonna be riding someone else's banana boat on your vacation.

You can help to avoid ED if you keep the meat out of your meat. If you eat a good vegetarian diet and exercise regularly, you'll have the stamina of a marathon runner. I mean, when was the last time your woman passed out from multiple orgasm exhaustion rather than boredom? Go meatless and become a sexual athlete with a black belt in Kama Sutra—not a chump who's stuck in that lame-ass missionary position.

All it takes to keep our schlongs happy and healthy

is the right balance of nutrients, minerals, and vitamins from organic, vegetarian food sources and regular exercise. There's a reason you feel like Joe Stud when you're working out. Your brain is releasing endorphins, your heart is pumping hard, your lungs are bringing in gulps of oxygen to allow your blood to flow freely, your libido is firing on all cylinders, and that fine-ass chick in spandex yoga pants is digging your shit . . . well, at least you can fantasize. Also, it should go without saying, but: Stop smoking! That shit went out in the eighties with cocaine and that Christian metal band Stryper. Smoking also reduces blood flow (among other things), so smoking doesn't make you a James Dean stud—it makes you a limp dick.

Nothing takes the magic out of your stick quicker than a poor diet and a sedentary lifestyle. If you spend your days eating shit food and sitting on your lazy ass in front of the TV, we need to talk. What chick would want to be with you for that ride? Maybe that poor little lady who signed on "in sickness and in health," but even wifey may leave your ass if you don't snap out of it. Trust me on that. Chicks like go-getters; the doers, not the talkers. About ten years ago the Physicians Committee for Responsible Medicine (PCRM) put out a hilarious ad titled "Room 103." The spot opens with a steamy sexual encounter that comes to a crashing halt. Wanna know what happened? The camera pans to the room service tray, where you see a fatty meat dinner.

Then the ad wraps up with a hard-hitting tagline: "Eating meat contributes to artery blockages—and that can make you impotent." PCRM nutrition director Amy Lanou has said, "Many middle-aged and older men are taking drugs like Viagra, not realizing the problem is their diet—loaded with saturated fat. Artery blockages don't just affect the heart. They can hit any organ." *Bingo!*

Jody Gorran, a fifty-three-year-old Florida business-man, encountered both ED and cardiovascular disease as a result of following the meat-heavy Atkins diet. Two years after beginning the diet, Gorran's health deteriorated to the point where he needed Viagra to maintain his manhood. Six months later, after developing a 99 percent blockage of a major coronary artery, he underwent his first angioplasty. Gorran says, "Erectile dysfunction was the least of my prob-lems. After my cardiac procedure, I refused to continue on the Atkins diet. I switched to a healthy, low–saturated fat diet. Within sixty days, my cholesterol level dropped from 215 to 146, and much to my surprise, I didn't need the Viagra anymore." Lanou backs up what Gorran's case sug-gests: "We encourage men experiencing ED and who are following any fatty diet—including Atkins—to switch to a low-fat, low-cholesterol vegetarian diet. It will help them lose weight healthfully and may also help them function better sexually."

Fellas, fuck the little blue pills. Grab your crotch, look

your dick in the eye, and repeat after me: "I will respect you. I will give you the proper foods, nutrition, and exercise you need to achieve maximum potential. I will never, ever clog you up with shitty food or cigarettes again." Now, let go of your junk and take back the control of your dick.

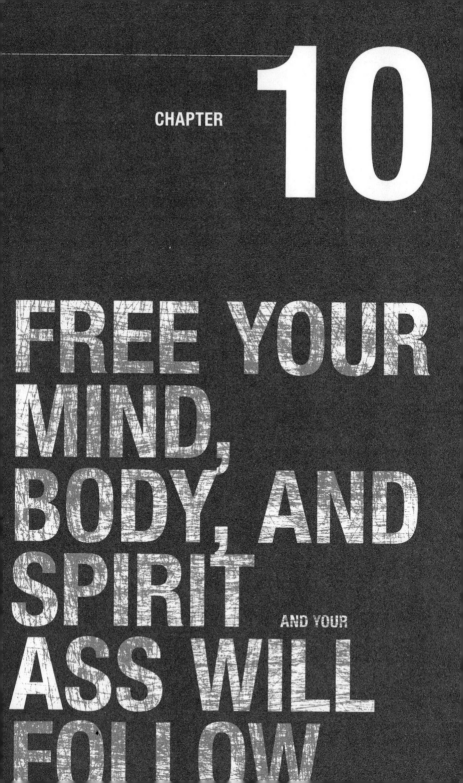

CHAPTER **10**

FREE YOUR MIND, BODY, AND SPIRIT AND YOUR ASS WILL FOLLOW

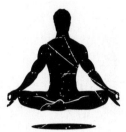

FREE YOUR MIND, BODY, AND SPIRIT AND YOUR ASS WILL FOLLOW

Now we've reached the part of the book that you knew was coming. It's no secret that becoming healthy requires a commitment to exercising—and that means you need to stop being a lazy pussy. I don't care how much healthy food you eat; if you don't exercise, you're going to gain weight. And for those of you who train and eat shit foods, it's time to start thinking about how your choices will affect you down the road because I can guarantee you with 100 percent certainty that they will.

The idea is to make fitness part of your lifestyle so you can be healthy and active into your fifties, sixties, and beyond. Everyone is different, though, and that's why I suggest you try a variety of things until you find the one you enjoy and can stick with. Maybe some of you guys are already cock-diesel gym rats and just need help with changing bad eating habits. Rock on, brothers; you'll find plenty of delicious options later in the book.

On the other hand, if you haven't been to the gym in a while (or ever) and just can't seem to get over the hump, I'm going to tell you what worked for me. And why should you listen to what I have to say? Well, at one point after a serious back injury and a bad relationship I fattened up to almost two hundred fucking pounds. At five foot nine, I looked and felt like shit. I was almost forty pounds over-weight and my super-athletic lifestyle was dead. When I hit a wall and crashed mentally, physically, and spiritually, eating became my only pleasure. I had to fight back. I had to start from day one.

That's the difference between "Someday" motherfuck-ers and "Day Oners"—Day Oners assign a task and start. Somedayers just keep putting it off . . . "Someday I'll get back in shape." Yeah, someday I'll fly to fucking India, too, but only if I buy a ticket, home slice. So with that being said before we get into our 30-Day Power Plan, let's address some very important issues so there are no stumbling blocks on your path.

THE MIND

——

Let's try a little exercise to see where your head is. As you read this, sit back and try to stop all the flowing rivers of bullshit that enter and exit your mind. Take some deep, slow breaths and listen to your body. Now, ask yourself what you're on earth to do. What is your purpose?

Maybe your purpose is to make a lot of money. Well, that's temporary, and you can't take it with you. Bang a lot of chicks? That's shallow, and everyone I know who does that ends up a lonely fucker with a bunch of STDs. Get that next job? Shit, that's no guarantee of success, as many of you nine-to-fivers well know.

Here's where I'm going with this: Slow down and take inventory. Life shouldn't be about all the bullshit we get caught up in every day. We're running like mindless idiots to our early graves. Do we really need every new gadget marketed to us? Every tantalizing food put in front of our faces? I mean, really, think about it.

A lot of people are unhappy or depressed because they listen to a bunch of A-holes who tell them how they're supposed to live. Depression never starts out full-blown; it creeps up, little by little. Drugs, alcohol, cigarettes, nutritional deficiencies, and lack of exercise all fuel depression and help it take hold. But I truly believe that purpose-driven people live a longer, happier, more ful-filling life, so let's make improving our well-being our primary purpose.

The reason we need to exercise our mind is simple: our mind can be our worst enemy or our best friend. The mind is a tool. Keep it engaged in positive things as much as possible and don't listen to it if it's telling you to get involved in nonsense. That's your enemy talking and your enemy will *never* tell you to do things that are beneficial for you. The mind controls the body, and if we aren't tough mentally, all of our desires to become fit will die in the road.

When I did my first Ironman in 2012 I had played a show with my band the night before in another city. I literally came offstage, got in my brother's car, drove back to New York, took a shower, and went to the swim start. I finished my race with *no sleep*. It was brutally hot, 93 degrees and humid. I remember tricking my mind the whole way through the 2.4-mile swim, 112-mile bike, and 26.2-mile marathon of hills. If it even hinted once at stopping I cursed it, "Shut the fuck up, you pussy motherfucker!" I'm not kidding you. People thought I was crazy because I was either cursing or chanting Hare Krishna the entire race.

My second Ironman in Mexico was just as harsh. I got my nose busted on the swim, my wetsuit tore and filled with water, and I had a stress fracture in my foot.

I was sunburnt to shit and bruised, but again I finished because I went into that tunnel where I was able to separate myself from the negative thoughts bubbling up in my mind. Eventually the stronger part of my mind just took over and made my body push on. But getting to that place only comes if you beat the mind with a stick on a daily basis.

The point is, what separates finishers from quitters in any aspect of life is that finishers know how to silence the mind when it kicks up those demons of doubt. If you can apply that discipline to this path of health and fitness you have a great shot at attaining the proper result.

Nine times out of ten it's not the task itself that kicks our asses, it's the attitude we approach that task with. I believe in approaching any situation with what I call a PMA: a positive mental attitude. Love what you are doing. Resistance loves a negative attitude, so don't let yourself go there. Watch your attitude and keep it in check. I learned that in 1980 from a Bad Brains song. They were the ones who were instrumental in my decision to go plant based and reverse my path of drugs, jails, and ultimately an early death.

"Don't care what they may say, we got that attitude, don't care what they may do, we got that attitude, hey we got that PMA."

They sang and I listened. You should, too.

THE BODY

———

Now that we've worked out our minds, we need to work out our bodies. The 30-Day Power Plan that follows will suggest, not dictate, things you can do to get into shape. Again, you need to discover what works best for you. But before you start an exercise program or take any natural supplements or minerals, make sure you check with your doctor. We don't want any bad interactions with any meds you're on now. Still, remember that my goal is to get you off those drugs and tell your pharmacist to fuck off . . . in a polite way, of course. (And to the crowd who think they can't afford to eat healthy but then spend half their paychecks on meds every month: please wake the fuck up and stop making excuses.)

First off, I like to get my metabolism going with some exercise *before* I eat breakfast. You're probably thinking, "What? Are you fucking crazy?" No, I'm not. It's just your weak-ass mind saying, "Eat! You need food the second you wake up!" NEWS FLASH: You don't. That's just the awful advice of your enemy mind.

Don't get me wrong. I'm not suggesting you embark on a fifteen-mile run or spend three hours in the gym. I'm talking about some yoga, a few push-ups, sit-ups, and pull-ups, a half-hour bike ride, a light jog, or maybe some rebounding. You ever see those mini trampolines? Those are called rebounders, and everyone should own one. Rebounding is a great cardio workout: rebounders aren't expensive and they don't take up a lot of space. Rebounding is low impact on the joints, and it burns plenty of calories. I strongly recommend Needak brand rebounders.

What you should eat and how much of it you should eat depends on your level of activity. Everything is according to time and circumstance. I've become an expert at listening to what my body is telling me. Eating the right foods in the right amounts at the right times plays just as big a part in my health as exercising does. In general you should aim to eat smaller, nutrient-dense meals throughout the day and consume a plant-based protein meal one to two hours after exercising.

When you starve yourself you tend to overeat, and when you skip meals like breakfast your metabolism slows down to conserve energy. The body is like a high-performance car. Put the right fuel in and you'll have the boost you need; put the wrong shit in and your body is sure to break down. But balance is the key. I use the acronym KISS—Keep It Simple, Stupid. A wise man shared it with me many years ago, and I've followed his advice ever since. You see, there's no need to overcomplicate things and write out a fucking schematic for every calorie and meal you consume. Yes, by all means keep a journal, that's important, but don't become a macro-psychotic, please, I beg of you. The world just doesn't need any more of those maniacs.

One of my major rules is that we shouldn't eat before bed. When you do that, your body stays up all night working to digest your food, and that takes energy. As a result, you don't give your body a chance to fully rest, restore, and repair—which is what sleep is meant to do. All of that digesting interferes with your sleep patterns. And because the excess food rests in your stomach, it causes pressure on the lower back area. Plus eating at night—when you're not going to be burning much energy—usually leads to weight gain. A lot of people I know who eat before bed have developed those great love handles. Who the hell loves those? You have to get proper rest as part of your new health regimen or you will crash and burn.

Buying healthy foods is only the first step. Being able to prepare, cook, and eat your own foods completes the process. The first step in healthy cooking is to throw away all of your aluminum pots and pans. Shitcan all that unnatural, chemical-laden nonstick crap, too. Use cast-iron pots, and pans. They last forever, hold heat, and cook food evenly, but most important, they release valuable iron into our food. When cooking vegetables, be careful not to overcook your food—when you cook plants for too long, they lose a lot of their nutrient value. Lightly sautéing or steaming veggies will keep their phytonutrients intact.

THE SPIRIT

———

Look, man, I'm not trying to fix your aura or make you wear tie-dye here. But I do feel that we, the human male species, have evolved enough to grasp the concepts I'm about to drop. Well, I hope that's the case, because chicks dig a dude who's in touch with his spiritual side. As a matter of fact, yoga spots and vegetarian restaurants are some of the best places to meet smoking-hot chicks who actually have some substance.

Now, think about this: if you do everything to take care of your body and don't pay attention to the spirit—the energy within the body that represents who we really are—then your search for happiness will remain incomplete. You'll always feel like you're missing something in your life. As a result, you'll look outside yourself for the next quick fix, that next magic bullet that promises to cure all. That's why people succumb to drugs and alcohol. I did.

Here's a pretty simple analogy for you: What if you had a pet bird but only took care of the cage? You clean it, hang jewelry on it, polish it, and so on, but never tend to the needs of the bird that lives inside it. See my point? The Vedas, which translates as "the knowledge," are a collection of ancient Indian texts. Among other spiritual offerings, they serve as the basis for all yogic philosophy. The texts teach us that the spirit controls our ego, our intelligence, our mind, our five senses, and ultimately our body. Nothing in this material world could exist without the presence of the spirit, which is our life force. The spirit is what gives us our individuality; it's what attracts people to each other. And if we choose not to embrace it, our body becomes an unattractive lump of shit. I mean, who the fuck wants to hook up with a dead body . . . aside from those necrophiliac fuckers?

As you start to appreciate the value of your spirit, you become more focused on your mission in life. You become less neurotic and understand that anything good takes time. That's why the first teaching in yoga is to meditate on the phrase "Aham Brahmasmi," which means "I am spirit."

Doing so offers a fresh perspective on life. Every living thing has its own spirit, so what right do we have to infringe on its life? You don't have the right to kill an animal because you feel like eating or wearing it. And if you don't think destroying billions upon billions of animals each year isn't affecting the global collective karma, you need to have your fucking head examined. You want peace, but where's the peace for them? The truth is that we've made this planet a hell for animals. Take a second, put yourselves in their place, and think about what we subject them to. It is hell.

When you think in terms of spirit, you stop seeing people as black or white, women or men. You have more respect toward all life. This is the real solution to war, racism, sexism, speciesism. My guru, A. C. Bhaktivedanta Swami Prabhupada, says that as long as people are in the bodily concept of life, there has to be conflict. We can't have real unity and equal rights on this planet until we embrace our spirit and start seeing everyone as equals.

I've seen people do some amazing things in life because they tapped into the energy of the soul, their spirit, the essence of who and what we *all* are. I can speak from my own experience. I was granted the gift of knowledge. If I had not had that chance I would not be writing this book, trust me. I probably wouldn't even be alive. Every day is a struggle, but as they say, I take it one day at a time.

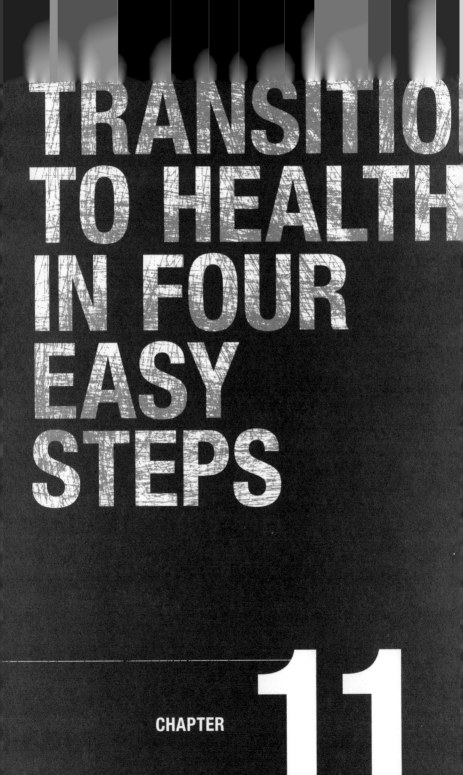

TRANSITION TO HEALTH IN FOUR EASY STEPS

CHAPTER 11

TRANSITION TO HEALTH IN FOUR EASY STEPS

1. USE STREET SMARTS

There are a lot of people out there in the field of medicine with fancy credentials who don't know shit about how to get you healthy. And there are others who are virtually on the pharmaceutical industry payroll, so all they do is write you prescriptions for another expensive drug.* Well, I'd love to meet these pricks face-to-face, but since that will probably never happen I've tried to do the next best thing, which is to warn you of the dangers and give you the advice that's worked for me all these years.

We have to see past the Great Food Bamboozle. The hoodwinkers in Big Pharma are in bed with them. You think Pfizer and the rest don't love McDonald's, Burger King, Pepsi, Cheetos, and KFC? When you go to the doctor for a minor ailment and he hands you a prescription, use that Stop and Think Mechanism. Should you stop eating Super Value Meals and drinking Big Gulps, or take some medicine to manage your pre-diabetes? You had better analyze and recognize.

2. TURN THE CORNER WITH DETOXIFICATION

Sometimes people who stop eating a poisonous diet consisting of meat, dairy, fish, processed foods loaded with toxic

---

* Think that's bullshit? Read the stunning book *Confessions of an Rx Drug Pusher*, by Gwen Olsen. The author, a former pharmaceutical executive, exposes the scumbag practices of doctors who receive payoffs and expensive gifts from pharmaceutical companies in exchange for prescribing dangerous, even deadly drugs to their patients. Drugs that some didn't even need.

preservatives, hydrogenated oils, and the rest of the bad shit, and start eating healthier, actually get sick at first. They assume that it is because of their new diet. They say stuff like, "I tried it and felt like shit." What's really going on is that the body is detoxifying itself. So, sure, you might feel run down, get some acne, maybe fevers and the runs, but it will pass, trust me. You've been poisoning yourself most of your life, and your body needs some time to clean house.

Here are a few things that might speed up the process: get colonics, drink an ounce or two of wheatgrass juice daily, try a short green-juice fast, and stick to raw foods for a little while. Also, remember to drink plenty of filtered water to flush the toxins out of your body. Let your blood, colon, and internal organs cleanse. Don't panic and flip out. Usually within a couple of weeks you'll start to feel better. Transition gradually. We never want to retreat in this war to take back our health.

3. KEEP ELIMINATING THE SHIT

There are so many hidden dangers slipped into our food without our knowledge it's un-fucking-believable. They even manage to shoot radiation into our food, spices, and herbs in a process called "irradiation." So always buy organic. Any doubt, leave it out. If you can't even pronounce the shit on the label, it shouldn't be in your body.

Here's what I want you to do. Every time you're about to buy something, break out your smartphone and do a little research. Go onto the Internet and see exactly what it is, where it came from, what the ingredients are, and how it was put into our food supply in the first place. (I would recommend doing the same thing with all personal hygiene and cleaning products as well.) I guarantee you that if you take the time to investigate what you're buying, you will not eat most of the shit you find at the grocery store.

Here is a list of food additives to avoid completely. If you see these on any food label, put it back on the shelf and run, don't walk, away.

THE SHIT LIST

———

Aspartame (chemical artificial sweetener)
MSG (labeled as flavorings)
high-fructose corn syrup (GMO)
rBGH (growth hormone in meat and dairy that'll get the fellas man-boobs and the ladies beards)

all refined and hydrogenated oils (trans fats)

BHA

BHT

sodium nitrates

fluoride

potassium bromate

propyl gallate

saccharin

olestra

artificial colorings

sulfites

refined sugars

sodium chloride

I can be here for days with this. The point I'm making: stop eating fucking processed food!

4. SUPERFOODS MAKE SUPERHUMANS

The term *superfood* is thrown around a lot lately. I've even heard people refer to beef and milk as "superfoods." They are not. Real superfoods are 100 percent non-animal and organic. Things like berries, nuts, seeds, fruits, vegetables, leafy greens, legumes, grains like quinoa, steel-cut oats, and amaranth. There are also a few items that I have added to my diet over the years that have amazing healing and nutritional properties. Again, do your own investigating, try things out, and see what you like.

THE DIRTY DOZEN

So you're eating more fruits and veggies and you're on the right path. Good for you, but not so fast, Slick. In order to really kick it up a notch these twelve should always be bought organically, as they have the heaviest amount of pesticide residue and the soil they were grown in is loaded with chemical fertilizers.

apples	strawberries
celery	kale
spinach	blueberries
peaches	cucumbers
nectarines	lettuce
potatoes	grapes

FAVORITE SUPERFOODS

Wheatgrass juice: One ounce of wheatgrass offers the equivalent of 2.5 pounds of green vegetables in nutritional value. It is a powerful thyroid stimulator, and because of its remarkable similarity to our own blood composition, regular consumption has tremendous anti-aging benefits.

Chia seeds: In pre-Columbian times chia seeds were a main component of the Aztec and Mayan diets and were the basic survival ration of Aztec warriors. They are rich in omega-3 fatty acids, protein, fiber, calcium, magnesium, iron, zinc, and antioxidants. They are also very good for diabetics because they regulate the speed at which sugar enters the bloodstream.

Goji berries: These delicious, low-calorie berries help to strengthen your immune system, increase energy, and curb cravings. They have one of the highest antioxidant contents in all foods and are a complete protein source. They also contain twenty-one trace minerals, more iron than spinach, and more vitamin C than an orange.

Flaxseed: Some call it one of the most powerful plant foods on the planet. There's some evidence that flaxseed may help reduce your risk of heart disease, cancer, stroke, and diabetes. Flaxseed contains omega-3 essential fatty acids,

MEAT IS FOR PUSSIES

"good" fats that have been shown to have heart-healthy effects; lingans, which have antioxidant qualities; and fiber.

Spirulina: Now considered one of the most nutritious food sources known to man. Spirulina was once called "the best food for the future" by the United Nations World Food Conference. This blue-green alga is a complete protein, rich in B vitamins, and has been reported to help correct anemia, reduce radioactive damage, and lower cholesterol.

Chlorella: This single-celled green alga is a powerhouse of nutrition. Extremely high in chlorophyll and magnesium, chlorella is a great detoxifier. Chlorella is also a complete protein source and aids in clear skin, blood sugar balance, mental clarity, digestion, and immune health.

Sprouted brown rice protein: This highly digestible, hypoallergenic, plant-based protein contains 83 percent protein derived from raw, sprouted whole-grain brown rice and is rich in vitamins, minerals, and amino acids. This form of protein is ideal for building lean muscle mass.

Blue-green algae: AFA (aphanizomenon flos-aquae) is one of nature's most efficient, versatile, and prolific nutritional powerhouses. AFA contains the highest known concentration of natural vegetable protein (58 percent) in the world as well as all of the essential amino acids in a perfect balance for the human body. Blue-green algae provides energy for life, mental clarity, and increased physical stamina. I use E3

Live and I swear by it. I get it in frozen form at the health food store and you can also find it at many juice shops.

Ginseng: This herb has been used for thousands of years to improve overall health and is specially recommended for increasing energy, reducing stress, and preventing illness. Always buy organic since ginseng farmers tend to use heavy pesticides and fungicides.

Maca: A root native to the high Andes of Peru, maca is a powerful adaptogen that works with the body to stabilize hormones and increase libido and energy, increasing oxygen uptake and endurance. Maca root also possesses natural means of improving sexual performance and has been referred to as "nature's Viagra."

Hemp seeds: Sorry, potheads, if you thought you could get high and get some protein, not with these. But hemp seeds not only are rich in omega-3 fatty acids but are a very good source of plant-based proteins as well. Three tablespoons of hemp seeds provide 16 grams of protein.

Lecithin: A fatty substance that is derived from plant tissues (it is also contained in egg yolks) and is a great source of choline, which is vital for brain function. It helps to break up cholesterol in the body and supports organ health, including the brain, heart, liver, and kidneys. Lecithin also contains inositol, which can aid in fat burning. I put two tablespoons in my shakes almost every day. Use only non-GMO formulas.

Turmeric: This bright yellow spice common in Indian cuisine has long been used as a powerful anti-inflammatory and has been effective in treating weak bones, soothing menstrual difficulties and bruises, as well as aiding in digestive relief. Studies have also shown turmeric to help prevent cancer and Alzheimer's disease, and to be effective in pain relief for arthritis.

So there you have it. Optimal health and studhood are within your reach. Four easy steps. You can do it.

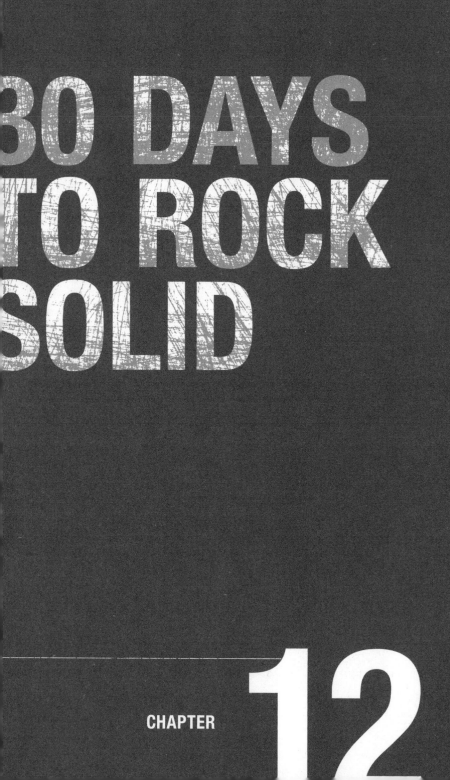

30 DAYS
TO ROCK
SOLID

CHAPTER 12

30 DAYS TO ROCK SOLID

*The Supercharged Path to Transform You into
One of the Fittest Humans on Two Legs*

These days everyone is talking about the obesity crisis. You hear that redundant phrase "the battle of the bulge" tossed around a lot. Bulge? It seems the more accurate phrase would be "battle of the behemoths." Take a walk down any street in America—I promise you, you're seeing a lot more than a few "bulges." Dig these numbers on the percentages of obesity by state:

Mississippi: 34.6%
Louisiana: 34.7%

West Virginia: 33.8%
Alabama: 33%

. . . and the list goes on and on.[38]

We're evolving into a new species, one I call *Ginormous homoerectus*. Darwin must be rolling over in his grave. When future inhabitants of planet earth dig up the ice and find preserved carcasses of a family of four, they're gonna need a fucking dump truck to haul them off to the Smithsonian.

So let's get down to business. Here's my challenge to all of you who want to lose weight. Just for right now, forget everything you think you know about diet and weight loss, and do what follows in this plan. Don't think about it, just do it. Exercise the way my man Aaron Drogoszewski (who has trained pro athletes like Reggie Bush, Carmelo Anthony, and Justin Tuck) tells you and utilize the amazing plant-based recipes you'll find in chapter 13. What do you have to lose?

I've been around a lot of badass people when it comes to training. One thing they all have in common is that they are consistent in their efforts and their discipline. They show up every day, *especially* the times when they didn't want to. But a lot of people—you know you've seen them—start working out with what I refer to as "the spring bee mentality." They're the ones who come buzzing around in May like, "It's springtime, yippee! Time to get a six-pack for the beach!" They show up at the gym for a month or two and then by September . . . hasta la vista, baby. They've either injured themselves from going all Joe Commando or just reverted to their laziness and bad habits. Don't be that guy.

We will cover all the bases. Leave no stones unturned. I even offer a Mental Toughness Training Tip (MTT) for the entire 30-Day program from myself as well as some of my amazing friends. These guys are at the top of their game—UFC fighters, Special Forces soldiers, active-duty Navy SEALs, and more. These people were all able to smash mental blocks and resistance and accomplish truly astounding things in their lives. Everyone gets tested, and everyone has setbacks along the way, even the above-mentioned badasses. I believe that without being tested you can never advance to the next level. But the philosophy behind this book and this fitness program is not about staying in neutral—hell fucking no. It's about constant and relentless forward motion to achieve your goal.

AARON'S FOUR GUIDING PRINCIPLES

The plan that follows is based on four guiding principles. These are the golden rules. Read them now, before you get started, and refer to them often as you progress through your workouts. They will keep you moving forward, and they will keep you honest.

1. ESTABLISH SMART GOALS

New Yorkers do not pay cabdrivers for the pleasure of their company, or so they can sit in the backseat and take in the scenery. Likewise, your fitness routine shouldn't just be simply about the journey, or the act of working out. Remember, whether it's with your money or with your time: you're paying for your fitness! Set goals for yourself that are Specific, Measurable, Accurate, Realistic, and Timely (SMART) to gauge your progress as you go along. "I want to get in shape" doesn't cut it. Round is a shape. Establish a four- to six-week goal with a realistic benchmark to measure against.

2. YOU CAN'T FIRE A CANNON FROM A CANOE

The typical resistance-training program often consists of movements engaging major muscle groups with very little focus on the muscles that stabilize them. While someone may have the ability to bench-press 225 pounds for fifteen repetitions, the bench on which they are performing that movement completely eradicates the necessity for the legs, glutes, or spinal stabilizers to support it. The only way this "strength" will ever translate outside the gym is when one is backed against a wall and needs to push something away. Let's keep our fingers crossed that none of the readers of this book ever find themselves in that particular scenario. You want to train the human movement system as a whole to develop your stabilization along with the major muscle groups.

3. DEDICATE MORE TIME TO TRAINING WEAKNESSES THAN STRENGTHS

Just because you walked through the gym doors doesn't mean you really showed up for your workout. If you're only doing the movements that you already feel confident with, you're not going to see the kind of improvements you're looking for. It's essential to spend your time wisely and keep yourself challenged physically, mentally, and emotionally— even if that means being uncomfortable with something new. When physical challenges are accepted, the gains made will transcend far beyond the walls of the gym.

4. UNDERSTANDING *CAN'T* VERSUS *WON'T*

Having a physical inability such as an injury that prevents you from conquering a challenge is acceptable. This happens in life and at the gym. These are the situations where you "can't" overcome the presented obstacle at the moment. It is not that you can't *ever* do it; it is about stopping to objectively dissect and understand *what* the problem is

MEAT IS FOR PUSSIES

and *where* it resides. For example, is the problem that you don't have enough endurance for a particular task? Is that a physical problem or is it in your head? Did you not eat enough or sleep enough? Breaking down the problem into a series of smaller variables helps you analyze and interpret your physical and mental skills and provides a tremendous opportunity for growth.

However, when the inability to overcome a challenge rests upon a foundation of self-doubt, focus on peripheral or emotional factors—this is a "won't." You can't get better when you "won't" take on a challenge. That's when my mental toughness tips come in. These are words and insights from some of the most badass people I know, and the goal is to use them as a tool to help you stay motivated every single day of the week. That means every time you're tempted to pussy out of a workout, or eat a McFat Burger instead of a plant-based, nutritious meal, check yourself with the words of people who actually walk the walk and don't make excuses.

That's it—those are the four commandments of this plan. They're simple, but important, so don't ignore them. Now, in closing here, let me reiterate that there are going to be people who will ridicule you for what you are undertaking, who tell you that you are eating or working out the wrong way. Most of the time, one look at them will be evidence enough not to listen to any of their unsolicited advice. You've gotta just let these idiots talk and keep going ahead with your bad self.

THE 411 ON 4/2/1

The majority of neuromuscular adaptations in muscular stabilization training made during the eccentric and isometric phases of contraction. In other words, when building a strong, stable foundation for physical fitness, it is most advantageous to stress the eccentric, or "negative," phase wherein the muscle is lengthened. This portion of the movement is given priority with a four-second count. Second priority is given to the isometric portion, or the "hold," with a two-second count. Coming in last is the concentric phase, or muscle shortening (the push in "push" movements, or the pull in "pull" movements), which is performed at a one count.

And, speaking of talk, I'm done here. So as we say on the mean streets of New York, it's time to put up or shut up. Let's do this. Yo, Aaron!!!!!

WHO IS THIS DUDE WHO'S TELLING ME WHAT TO DO?

Aaron Drogoszewski is the trainer who got me ready to tackle my Ironman triathlons. I had some pretty serious old injuries when we started working together but he got me through them, and today I feel fitter and stronger than ever. He's legit. And he has a resume to prove it.

CERTIFICATIONS:

- NASM Master Instructor
- API Caveman Master Instructor
- NASM CPT
- NASM CES
- NASM PES
- NASM MMACS
- NASM FNS
- KBA Level 1 Kettlebell Coach
- DVRT Sandbag Level 1 Coach
- TRX Suspension
- USA Boxing Level 1 Coach
- Black Belt Okinawan Goju Ryu
- Two-time New York City Golden Gloves "Fighter of the Night"
- Muay Thai Kickboxer
- Purple Belt Brazilian Jiujitsu

CELEBRITIES HE'S WORKED WITH:

- Reggie Bush
- Justin Tuck
- Carmelo Anthony
- Arian Foster
- Sam Rockwell
- Matt Damon
- Paul Schneider
- Penn Badgley
- Chris Messina
- "Irish" Micky Ward
- Maureen "the real million-dollar baby" Shea
- Peter "Kid Chocolate" Quillin
- Deontay Wilder (Olympic bronze medalist boxer)

FITNESS EVALUATION

Before you get started, we're going to have you take a test to determine what level of fitness you're at now. Below is a circuit of exercises that make up the test. Be sure to perform each exercise with a full range of motion and proper form. Run through these at a fast yet controllable pace—you are competing against yourself. Here are the rules:

- Record how long it takes you to complete this circuit two days before beginning the 30-day challenge.
- Retest for evaluation two days after you complete the 30-day challenge.
- Perform the movements in identical fashion for both attempts to ensure accurate results.

THE CIRCUIT:
- 100 rotations with jump rope
- 10 push-ups
- 10 alternating reverse lunges with each leg (20 lunges total)
- 10 stationary squat jumps
- 100 rotations with jump rope
- 5 push-ups
- 6 alternating reverse lunges with each leg (12 lunges total)
- 5 squat jumps
- 100 rotations with jump rope
- 10 push-ups

- 10 alternating reverse lunges with each leg (20 lunges total)
- 10 stationary squat jumps

FITNESS GLOSSARY AND HOW-TO

You're going to need to know a few terms to complete this 30-day cycle. None of the exercises here are rocket science, but if you haven't worked out in a while, the names of the movements might be new to you. Here's a cheat sheet you can refer to as you go through the plan. I'm just covering the basics here. You have any questions—don't hurt yourself, look it up. There are thousands of websites that can walk you through this stuff with videos.

STRENGTH TRAINING TERMINOLOGY

Push-ups
Keep your back flat by drawing in your belly button to spine as tight as possible, glutes contracted (think about holding something between your butt cheeks as hard as possible) for entire movement. You want to

aim for a 4/2/1 tempo= 4 seconds to lower from arms-extended position to floor; 2-second hold 2 inches from the ground; 1-second extension away from floor to starting position.

Modification: When unable to perform push-ups with proper form, modify by placing hands on a stable table, bench, or wall with feet on the floor (so you are at approximately a 45-degree angle or taller). This will decrease the necessity for core stabilization and will keep the whole body active. Placing knees on the floor is acceptable, but not ideal.

Cobras

Lying facedown with a neutral curve through spine, and face/chest 1–2 inches from the ground, with both arms extended to the sides of the body and palms touching the ground, contract quads and glutes.

Squeeze shoulder blades together and down toward hips (do not allow shoulders to elevate toward the ears), rotating arms and thumbs away from the body and toward the ceiling (thumbs leave the ground first, before pinky finger).

Aim for 4/2/1 tempo: 1-second contraction of shoulder blades and elevation of chest from floor; 2-second hold at peak with shoulder blades contracted and thumbs rotated; 4-second return to facedown starting position.

Single-leg T's

Stand on one leg in a "tabletop" position, bent over at the waist with a neutral curve through spine so the back/chest is parallel to the floor.

With arms extended toward the floor, thumbs turned out away from center of body/palms forward, bring both arms up toward ceiling until parallel to the floor, with arms creating a T shape with spine and shoulders.

Maintain tabletop position for entire set.

Aim for 4/2/1 tempo= 1-second contraction from bottom starting position to T shape; 2-second hold at peak of T; 4-second return from T to bottom/starting position.

Reverse lunge to balance

Start with both feet hip width apart with insides of feet parallel to one another. Step back with the right leg to lunge position, with forward angle of the back creating a parallel line between spine/left shin. Keep your left foot flat on the ground (do not allow heel to elevate). The majority of your weight is distributed through left/front leg with arms lowered toward the foot of left/front leg. Keep shoulders pulled back and do not round middle of the back.

Driving strictly through left/front leg, extend to standing position with right/back foot off the floor with right knee drawn to waist height.

Alternate legs, or continue same side as indicated.

Aim for a 4/2/1 tempo = 4 seconds to lower to bottom of lunge "runner's start"; 1-second extension to single-leg balance position; 2-second hold at single-leg balance position with proper posture.

Squat jump to stabilization

Start with feet hip width apart, and insides of the feet parallel to one another.

Lower to squat position, keeping weight distributed over the entire foot, hips stuck out slightly behind the heels, neutral spine, and knees tracking over (never inside of) the second and third toes (think of sitting down into a chair).

Jump while extending knees completely, and toes toward the floor to a height conducive to landing quietly and smoothly back to starting position (do not allow knees to cave inside of second and third toes, or feet to turn out).

Hold squat for 3–5 seconds before continuing.

Variation: Lateral squat jumps: Follow instructions for squat jump while jumping side to side.

Variation: Rotational squat jumps: Follow instructions for squat jump while rotating 90–180 degrees with each jump.

CARDIOVASCULAR TERMINOLOGY

Zone 1

"Talk test": While in zone 1, you should feel as though you are working with an elevated heart rate, but be able to speak aloud *without* conflict, and in normal speech patterns (should be able to have a normal conversation with a friend working out next to you). At zone 1, you should be at 65–75 percent of your maximum perceived heart rate.

Zone 2

"Talk test": While in zone 2, you should feel as though you are working at a difficult yet controllable pace, and capable of speaking aloud *with* interruption (able to speak to a friend while working out, but with frequent gaps to take in deep breaths). At zone 2, you should be at 80–85 percent maximum perceived heart rate.

Zone 3

"Talk test": This is a maximum effort cardiovascular zone, wherein your workload and heart rate will be too high to be able to verbalize aloud with clarity (sprinting to the point where you are too out of breath to be able to speak to the friend next to you). At zone

3, you should be at 86–90 percent maximum perceived heart rate.

CIRCUIT TYPES

Horizontal Load Circuit

Completing all sets of an exercise for a given muscle group with prescribed rest between before moving on to the following movement/muscle group.

Vertical Load Circuit

Performing one set of an exercise for each muscle group provided in circuit fashion (moving with little to no rest from chest/back/shoulders/legs). You will typically have a longer rest time after a vertical load circuit, after which time you will start the circuit again.

THE 30-DAY POWER PLAN

WEEK 1

Monday/Wednesday/Friday: Resistance Training
The Workout: Horizontal load circuit
(Approximately 45 minutes)

12 push-ups
- 4/2/1 tempo
- 2 sets total
- 60 seconds rest between sets

15 floor cobras
- 4/2/1 tempo
- 2 sets total
- 60 seconds rest between sets

15 single-leg T's
- 4/2/1 tempo
- 2 sets total
- 60 seconds rest between sets

12–20 alternating reverse lunges
- 4/2/1 tempo
- 2 sets total
- 60 seconds rest between sets

MONDAY MTT TIP: "Mondays are a mother-fucker for some people. Not for me they ain't. For me it's another opportunity to chip away at my goal. So make sure you set one and keep that PMA. That's how I start my week off properly."

—JOHN J.

WEDNESDAY MTT TIP: "My clients know what I know: the more you move the less likely mental demons are to catch you."

—ORION MIMS, Finisher of 11 marathons, 16 half and 10 full Ironmans, also my Ironman coach

FRIDAY MTT TIP: "When you get tired and think you can't do another rep, that's when the real training starts. That's when you develop the mind/body connection to push through."

—ERIKA MITCHENER, NASM Certified Trainer, fitness model, and black belt

Tuesday/Thursday/Saturday: Reactive and Cardiovascular Training
(Approximately 50 minutes)

Stationary squat jump to stabilization
- 10 repetitions
- 3–5 seconds hold at stabilization
- 2 sets

- 60 seconds rest between sets

20–30 minutes zone 1 cardiovascular work

Personal preference of walking/running/jump rope

TUESDAY MTT TIP: "Set realistic goals and understand your limitations. That way on the days that are hard, you don't become overfrustrated and give up entirely. That way, your victories are that much sweeter when they come."

—ACTIVE-DUTY NAVY SEAL

THURSDAY MTT TIP: "You have to beat the mind with a stick every morning."

—A. C. BHAKTIVEDANTA SWAMI PRABHUPADA, my yoga teacher
and the toughest person ever!

SATURDAY MTT TIP: "Just start training; don't overthink it. Learn as you go and embrace the journey. Mood follows action, not the other way around."

—RICH ROLL, plant-based Ultraman and author of *Finding Ultra*

Sunday: Day off!

MTT TIP: "Take inventory of how you feel. Write it down. Keeping a journal doesn't make you a pussy; it makes you someone who is striving to get somewhere."
—JOHN J.

WEEK 2

Monday/Wednesday/Friday: Resistance Training
The Workout: Horizontal load circuit
(Approximately 45 minutes)

12–15 push-ups
- 4/2/1 tempo
- 3 sets total
- 60 seconds rest between sets

15–20 floor cobras
- 4/2/1 tempo
- 3 sets total
- 60 seconds rest between sets

15–20 single-leg T's
- 4/2/1 tempo
- 2 sets total
- 60 seconds rest between sets

12–20 reverse lunges
- 4/2/1 tempo

Complete 12–20 repetitions on first leg before alternating to opposite leg for 12–20 repetitions
2 sets total per leg
60 seconds rest between sets

MONDAY MTT TIP: "Right now is the time, the time to push. Push past what your mind says are your limits. That fatigue is Improvement. The struggle is the reward."

—TODD VANCE, Former Army Special Forces

WEDNESDAY MTT TIP: "Every day *you* have a choice, tough times hit everyone, what do you choose here, right now? . . . There is a reason eagles don't fly in flocks!"

—JON HINDS, Founder of the Monkey Bar Gymnasium (first plant-based gyms in the world!)

FRIDAY MTT TIP: "The first step to true mental toughness comes through emotional flexibility, giving yourself permission to feel scared, uncomfortable, or angry in the moment. Once permission is granted, and you learn how to harness your

fears, and utilize them, you are a weapon both in competition and in life."
—AARON DROGOSZEWSKI

Tuesday/Thursday/Saturday: Reactive and Cardiovascular Training
(Approximately 30–35 minutes)

10–15 lateral squat jumps to stabilization
- 3–5 seconds hold at stabilization
- 2 sets total
- 60 seconds hold between sets

Cardiovascular (preference of walk/run/jump rope)
5 minutes zone 1
1 minute zone 2
5 minutes zone 1
1 minute zone 2
5 minutes zone 1
1 minute zone 2
10 minutes zone 1

TUESDAY MTT TIP: "The enemy mind hates when you are organized and regimented, when you set a consistent routine and stick with it because it knows it will be defeated if you do that."

—JOHN J.

THURSDAY MTT TIP: "Mental toughness is much more important than the physical. Train your mind, stay focused, and attack your training as if you're a warrior."

—FRED BISCI

SATURDAY MTT TIP: "Do something that you find exciting, have the courage to pursue it, and also keep evolving."

—MIKE MAHLER, Plant-based strength coach and kettlebell instructor

Sunday: Day off!

MTT TIP: "Always remember the reason you are embarking upon this journey is to improve your health and there will be ups and downs, I guarantee you that. So monitor everything, even those shittiest of moments of mental resistance. Monitor, put them in check, and move the fuck on."

—JOHN J.

WEEK 3

Monday/Wednesday/Friday: Resistance Training
The Workout: Vertical load circuit
(Approximately 20 minutes)
0–30 seconds rest between movements
60 seconds rest upon completion of circuit
2 complete circuits total

12–20 push-ups
- 4/2/1 tempo

12–20 floor cobras
- 4/2/1 tempo

12–20 single-leg T's
- 4/2/1 tempo

12–20 alternating reverse lunges
- 4/2/1 tempo

MONDAY MTT TIP: "The body and mind work as one machine. I get rid of mental FEAR and then I'm able to put both to work for me."

—ANONYMOUS, world-class martial artist and senior agent, Diplomatic Security Service

WEDNESDAY MTT TIP: "The key to any great physical challenge is to constantly see yourself at the finish line, every single day. If the mind truly believes it the body will obey."

—FRANK GRILLO, Actor

FRIDAY MTT TIP: "Every man falls. Champions dust their ass off and keep fighting. A misstep is only a failure when you identify it as one. When you identify a misstep as an opportunity to evolve, the experience transforms to a rung in the ladder of your inevitable success."

—AARON DROGOSZEWSKI

Tuesday/Thursday/Saturday: Reactive Training and Cardiovascular Training
(Approximately 40 minutes)

Lateral squat jump to stabilization
- 10–12 repetitions
- 3–5 seconds hold at stabilization
- 1 set with 60 seconds rest before following movement

Rotational squat jump to stabilization
- 10–12 repetitions

- 3–5 seconds hold at stabilization
- 1 set with 60 seconds rest before following movement

Cardiovascular
5 minutes zone 1
1 minute zone 2
30 seconds zone 3
5 minutes zone 1
1 minute zone 2
30 seconds zone 3
5 minutes zone 1
1 minute zone 2
10 minutes zone 1

TUESDAY MTT TIP: "Every person I've ever met who accomplished amazing things in both life and fitness, those individuals who assign a task and obliterate it to fucking pieces all have one thing in common . . . they never let mental resistance stop them."

—JOHN J.

THURSDAY MTT TIP: "Fatigue makes cowards of us all. Eat plant-strong and train consistently and you'll be able to push yourself past mental blocks to the next level while others fall off the back."

—RIP ESSELSTYN, FORMER FIREFIGHTER, Author of *The Engine 2 Diet*

SATURDAY MTT TIP: "Self-talk, meditation, even prayer or self-reflection helps you find your way through a lot of the hard times. If you can talk yourself through it, you can make yourself do it."

—ACTIVE-DUTY NAVY SEAL

Sunday: Day off!

MTT TIP: "Your goal is in sight, but never look back because the mind is a tricky fucker. It will tell you how great you've done, how far you've come, and that it's okay to call it a day. Always look ahead; that's where the finish line is."

—JOHN J.

WEEK 4

Monday/Wednesday/Friday: Resistance Training
The Workout: Vertical load circuit
(Approximately 30–35 minutes)
No rest between movements

60 seconds rest upon completion of circuit
3 complete circuits total

12–20 push-ups
- 4/2/1 tempo

12–20 floor cobras
- 4/2/1 tempo

12–20 single-leg T's
- 4/2/1 tempo

12–20 alternating reverse lunges
- 4/2/1 tempo

MONDAY MTT TIP: "Leave everything here in this cage, in the gym. All your hurt all your guilt all your regrets all your frustration. When you hit your wall, think of all that, and smash it! You can choose to step up to a challenge."

—TODD VANCE, Former Army Special Forces, POW, MMA head instructor

WEDNESDAY MTT TIP: "World-class athlete and Navy SEAL David Goggins said that when you think you're done and you can't go further you've only tapped into 40 percent of what you're capable of, the rest is in the mind."

—RICH ROLL, plant-based Ultraman and author of

Finding Ultra

FRIDAY MTT TIP: "Having a deep mental resistance to do something, especially getting in shape and watching what you eat, means there is a deep need for it."

—JOHN J.

Tuesday/Thursday/Saturday: Reactive and Cardiovascular Training

(Approximately 30–35 minutes)

Lateral squat jump to stabilization

- 12–15 repetitions
- 3–5 seconds hold at stabilization
- 1 set with 60 seconds rest before following movement

Rotational squat jump to stabilization

- 12–15 repetitions
- 3–5 seconds hold at stabilization
- 1 set with 60 seconds rest before following movement

Cardiovascular
5 minutes zone 1
30 seconds–1 minute zone 3
5 minutes zone 1
1 minute zone 2
5 minutes zone 1
30 seconds–1 minute zone 3
5 minutes zone 1
1 minute zone 2
5 minutes zone 1

TUESDAY MTT TIP: "I got serious about running because I like running. It's that simple. I do it because I want to. In the middle of a race, if my body feels like it's getting tired, I just ask myself, 'What would I rather be doing?' And the answer is always 'NOTHING.'"

—BRENDAN BRAZIER, Author of *Thrive*

THURSDAY MTT TIP: "The first time I made it to the finals of a tournament I was really tired. I started to worry. But when I looked across the mat I realized my opponent was tired too. Everyone gets tired. The ones who can stay composed and power through mentally . . . win."

—JOSH GRIFFITHS, Third-degree black belt in Brazilian jiujitsu

SATURDAY MTT TIP: "Mental toughness, just like muscles, can be trained. The key is to keep extending one's boundaries. It's about putting yourself in uncomfortable situations, testing your willpower, going a little further."

—JAMES "LIGHTNING" WILKS, UFC Ultimate Fighter champion

So you finished your first 30 days. Good—take a moment and pat yourself on the back because you deserve it. Now start another cycle. Add to the reps Aaron provided. Double them if you're feeling studly. Even try doing some two-a-days once or twice week. Cardio in the morning, resistance at night, switch it around, whatever. Always change your routine to avoid the plateau effect as well as mental boredom. Go join a gym, set a goal to do a 10K run, a marathon, a charity bike ride, a Spartan Death Race, whatever. Always set goals and work toward an objective; don't just float through your workouts or your life. You can either spend your time wisely or hang out in bars getting shit-faced, putting bad food in your gut, and playing video games. Your choice.

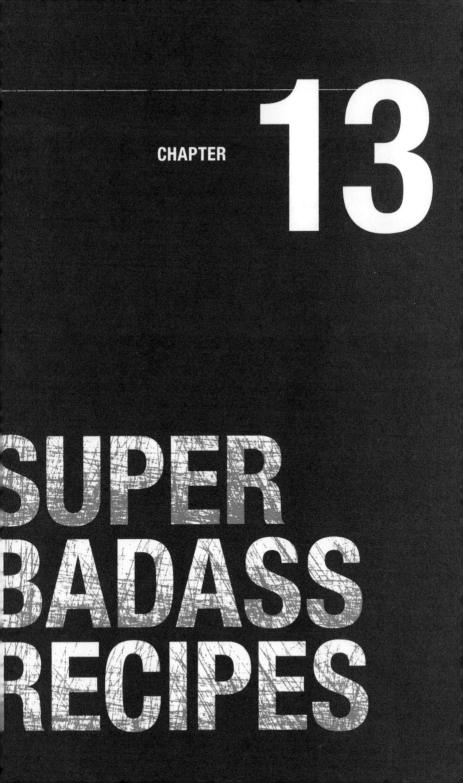

CHAPTER **13**

SUPER
BADASS
RECIPES

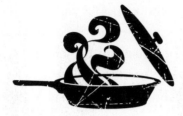

SUPER BADASS RECIPES

If we want to truly get healthy and fit, we have to feed our bodies the right fuel. In this chapter I'll give you a variety of plant-based and delicious options for every meal of the day, plus juices, shakes, and snacks. So there's plenty to work with here. Just see what's right for you and build your daily menu for 30 days.

You may have noticed that going plant based is one of the biggest trends in fitness circles nowadays. Everyone from pro boxers to Mixed Martial Arts fighters to professional football, baseball, and hockey players to triathletes is making the switch. So if you have any concerns that a plant-based diet won't give you the energy you need to do the workout program, you might want to consider that if it's good enough for elite athletes, it'll probably work for you, too. The days of fueling your workouts with steak and boiled chicken, whey protein, and raw eggs went out with tiger-striped gym pants. Remember Brendan Brazier's advice—eat carbs before exercising to give your body a simple energy source, and have some protein afterward to help build and repair muscle.

There are three appliances that I would suggest you invest in for your new, healthy kitchen: a juicer, a blender, and a dehydrator. I like to eat around my juicer, which means I drink a variety of fresh, organic, cold pressed veggie and fruit juices every day. If you don't want to spend the money on a juicer, you can use a blender for these recipes and just strain out the fruit and vegetable pulp (or leave it in if you like it—it's full of fiber). Food dehydrators have so many uses—you can dehydrate fruit and nuts, and even make kale chips—and it's super-easy. I like the Excalibur model and you can score a five-tray one for around $175. And as I mentioned earlier, a set of nontoxic cookware—ideally cast iron—is essential.

Also when it comes to investing in a healthy kitchen, I can't urge you enough to use organic ingredients even down to the spices, which should always be nonirradiated. Eating organic can be affordable if you buy in bulk and stick to a meal plan for the week. If you do buy nonorganic produce, make sure you stay away from the Dirty Dozen (see page 142).

The food you will be preparing is so rich in nutrients and fiber that you'll find yourself feeling full more quickly than you did when you ate junk. Processed foods have virtually no nutrients or fiber, which is why people tend to overeat them. Think about it—how easy is it to eat a whole bag of chips? But a bag of carrots? Celery? You couldn't make it halfway through without feeling stuffed. So you can either have an amazing plant-based gourmet meal or gorge yourself on a fast-food burger and fries that's going to make you feel lethargic and leave you hungry again in an hour. It's kind of a no-brainer, isn't it?

I've called upon some of my friends who are great cooks to share their best plant-based recipes with you. Whether you are just starting out and making the switch to a plant-based diet, or you're already a pro, there's something here for everyone. For me cooking is meditative. I love it and you will, too, once you grasp the basics. Always do the prep work and lay everything out first. You don't want chaos in the kitchen, chopping veggies and measuring once you have your fire going. I recommend doubling recipes and making more than you need whenever possible because you'll have leftovers on hand to bring to work, school, or an after-gym training session. Remember, if you fail to prepare, you prepare to fail, so don't get caught without a plan.

I don't snack while I'm cooking or sample the foods I'm prepping. Personally, I believe God (Krsna) puts all these wonderful things for us to eat here on earth. That's my thing. Therefore I feel it's important to recognize that and offer my food to God first. I try to cook in a loving way, as I'm actually cooking for God. When you cook like that the food becomes energized, and I have to tell you, me and my peeps have even gotten intoxicated with positive energy after eating food prepared that way. That's not some new-age crap, that's real talk from a real dude.

The best advice I can give you is to try these recipes, see what you like, what works in your busy day, what works for your budget, what your kids will eat—discover the best choices for all of your personal variables. I'm not here to tell you how to eat every single meal and morsel of food for the rest of your life like some OCD fucking lunatic nutritionist. I'm just here to offer you some knowledge and some options. That's half the battle—the other half is up to you. You have to invest the time to grocery shop, outfit your kitchen, and start cooking your own meals. So let's get busy.

BREAKFAST IDEAS

It's been said that breakfast is the most important meal of the day. I believe that every meal is important, but it is true that skipping breakfast causes your metabolism to crash and burn. Try some of these recipes to start your day out strong.

PROTEIN ENDURANCE SMOOTHIE
by Chef Pete Cervoni

Pete is a great friend and is currently the head chef at Organic Avenue, one of New York City's top plant-based destinations. His tip: for easier blending, you can place the dates in the filtered water and allow them to soak overnight in the refrigerator. When making the smoothie, use all the dates along with their soaking water. For a colder and thicker smoothie, you can replace one cup of the filtered water for 1½ cups of ice cubes.

Makes 2 quarts (approximately 4 servings)

6½ cups filtered water
3 cups dates, pitted
1 cup hemp seeds, shelled
1½ tbsps chia seeds
⅛ tsp (pinch) Himalayan pink salt
2 tablespoons lucuma powder
1 tbsp maca powder
½ cup cacao powder

2 tbsp sprouted brown rice protein
2 tbsp greens powder

Place all ingredients in a high-speed blender, such as a Vitamix, and process on high for 45–60 seconds until all the ingredients (especially the dates) have broken down completely and you achieve a rich and creamy shake. Serve immediately or store for up to three days in an airtight container, refrigerated.

ENERGIZING GREEN JUICE

Makes 2 servings

Sometimes I like to start my day off with a green juice. It sends your energy levels through the roof. Remember, juice oxidizes and loses potency with every passing minute so always drink your juice right away if possible. Never peel veggies; a lot of nutrients are in the skin. So just get an organic vegetable brush and clean them in water.

6 large carrots
1 apple, cut into eighths
1 sprig parsley
1 cup of spinach

3 celery stalks
½ cup beets

Add all ingredients to juicer, and enjoy your juice immediately, or store in the fridge in an airtight container and
consume within forty-eight hours.

SUPER POWER SHAKE

Makes 2 servings

We've all been there. Not enough time for a meal because
we got things to do. Don't sweat it. This amazing shake will
get you through anything the day throws at you. If you don't
have a high-end blender like a Vitamix or Omega, make sure
you don't overblend, as the blades of the cheaper models heat
up and destroy nutrients. I put my liquid in first and blend
with the spinach, then I add the other ingredients.

4 cups Living Harvest vanilla hemp milk (you can
substitute water if desired)
2 scoops Vega Berry Flavor Complete Whole Food
Optimizer
1 cup chopped spinach
1 scoop Sunwarrior brand Ormus Supergreens

½ cup chia seeds (soak in water and stir for 10
    minutes)
1 tbsp maca
1 tsp cinnamon
1 tbsp non-GMO lecithin granules
½ cup Brazil nuts (soaked in water overnight)
2 tbsp Udo's High Lignan loaded with omega oils
    3-6-9
1½ cups frozen blueberries (or other frozen berries)

Place all ingredients into the blender and blend until
combined into a thick, creamy shake. Serve immediately.

JOINT FIXER GREEN JUICE

Fresh pineapple is rich in bromelain, which is a complex
mixture of substances that can be extracted from the skin
and core fruit of the pineapple. So use a vegetable brush
and scrub the skin for extra nutrients. Bromelain is a serious anti-inflammatory, as are gingerroot and turmeric,
which makes this a great juice for when you experience
joint pain, headaches, or other inflammatory issues.

½ pineapple
4 stalks celery
1–2 cucumbers

3–4 leaves of red chard
small slice of ginger
¼ tsp turmeric powder

Place all ingredients into the juicer, except for the turmeric. Stir the turmeric into the finished juice. Enjoy your juice immediately, or store in the fridge in an airtight container and consume within forty-eight hours.

SKIN TRIP JUICE

Makes 2 servings

This juice is one of my favorites. It's great for the liver, blood, and skin. Always make juice 60–90 minutes before you eat. I always stagger carrots with other ingredients as they help flush everything out of your juicer. In other words, put in your beets and pare one carrot. Then your cucumber, dandelion, and another carrot, etc. Leave one carrot for the last thing going in.

6 medium carrots
1 pear
1 small beet—cut in eighths
1 large peeled cucumber (even organic has wax)

4 stalks celery
1 six-inch piece of aloe insides
Small piece gingerroot
6 leaves dandelion

Place all ingredients into the juicer. Enjoy your juice immediately, or store in the fridge in an airtight container and consume within forty-eight hours.

THE GREEN MONSTER

Makes 2 servings

This juice is loaded with nutrients and is alkalizing to the body. Acidity is your enemy—the Green Monster is the answer. Kale tends to be a little bitter, so if you want a sweeter juice, add a little more apple.

2 large carrots
1 large peeled cucumber
6 large kale leaves
½ cup spinach
4 stalks celery
½ cup alfalfa sprouts
½ lemon, peeled

1 apple

1 ounce of E3 Live (available in the frozen section of
many health food stores)

Place all ingredients into the juicer. Enjoy your juice immediately, or store in the fridge in an airtight container
and consume within forty-eight hours.

NUT-FREE TAHINI CHIA

by Chef Daniel Ceballos

Makes 2 8-oz servings

My friend Daniel Ceballos submitted this recipe. He is
the head chef at Juice Press in New York City and a very
grounded and spiritual cat. This makes a super-creamy,
satisfying shake that is an easy substitute for a meal.

1 cup filtered water

5 pitted medjool dates

½ cup raw tahini (substitute ½ cup soaked cashews if
desired)

⅛ cup chia

1 tsp vanilla extract

1 ripe mashed banana (optional)
pinch of sea salt
¼ tsp cinnamon

Put all ingredients in blender except for chia and mashed banana and blend well until creamy.

In a separate mixing bowl add chia and ¼ cup of filtered water and whisk briefly. Stir in the contents of the blender and mashed banana and mix thoroughly.

Allow to sit covered for 15–20 minutes. Serve with your favorite seasonal fruit or berries for a complete nutrient-dense and digestive-friendly meal.

TOASTED APPLE CINNAMON CEREAL

by Brendan Brazier

Makes 4 cups or about 5 servings

Brendan Brazier has kindly shared this one from his book, *Thrive Diet*. This is an excellent cereal in terms of nutritional balance. Unlike many commercial cereals, this one has lots of fiber, complete protein, essential fatty acids, and calcium.

½ apple, diced

1 cup oats (or cooked or sprouted quinoa to make
     cereal gluten-free)

½ cup diced almonds

½ cup ground flaxseed

½ cup hemp flour

½ cup unhulled sesame seeds

½ cup sunflower seeds

1½ tsp cinnamon

¼ tsp nutmeg

¼ tsp stevia

¼ tsp sea salt

¼ cup hemp oil

¼ cup molasses

2 tbsp apple juice

Preheat oven to 250° F.

Combine apple, oats, almonds, ground flaxseed, hemp flour, sesame seeds, sunflower seeds, cinnamon, nutmeg, stevia, and sea salt. Blend together hemp oil, molasses, and apple juice. Combine liquid and dry ingredients and mix well. Spread on a baking tray lightly oiled with coconut oil. Bake for 1 hour. Let cool, then break into pieces. Store refrigerated in an airtight container for up to two weeks.

TOFU SCRAMBLE WITH BREAKFAST SAUSAGE

Makes 4–6 servings

This is a great substitute for those nasty sausage and egg breakfasts that'll clog your arteries and zap your energy. I always make extra in case I want to whip up a breakfast burrito the next day. Make sure you get non-GMO soy sausage with no egg whites (Field Roast is a great brand). Throw the soy sausage in a hot cast-iron skillet with a teaspoon of coconut oil, asafetida, and black pepper. Make sure you roll them in the spices to pick up the flavor. Sear them on all sides until they're golden brown. Don't overcook; they suck when they get dry.

> 3 tbsp coconut oil
> 2 packets Fantastic Tofu Scrambler Seasoning Mix
> 2 1-lb blocks extra-firm tofu, mashed really well
> 1 cup broccoli florets
> 2 cups baby spinach, washed and stemmed
> 1½ cups cauliflower, cut into florets
> ½ cup sliced green zucchini
> ½ cup unsalted artichoke hearts
> ½ cup chopped red bell peppers
> ½ cup raw cashew pieces
> 1 tbsp black mustard seeds

2 tsp cumin powder

1 tsp fenugreek seeds

1 tsp hing (aka asafetida)

1 tsp turmeric

pinch of garam masala

pinch of black pepper

1 tbsp sea salt (more if you need it, less if you need
    low sodium)

2 dried red chili peppers

1 cup Daiya cheddar cheese (optional)

½ cup plain coconut yogurt

Heat oil in a cast-iron skillet and add the chili peppers. Let them fry for 30 seconds and add mustard seeds. When mustard seeds begin to crackle, add fenugreek seeds, turmeric, hing, cumin powder, garam masala, black pepper, and salt. Let spices fry for 45 seconds as you stir them around. Now add cauliflower and cashews and sauté for one minute over a medium flame. Then add all veggies except spinach and stir and cover. Sauté on medium flame for 5 minutes.

Once the veggies are slightly tender, add Tofu Scrambler mix, tofu, and one tablespoon of water. Stir everything together and cook for 7 minutes. Add spinach and stir. Once everything is all together, add cheese and allow to melt.

Top individual portions with yogurt.

To make a sweet tofu scramble wrap, preheat your oven to 350° F. Grab a wrap (Food For Life, Rudi's, and Ezekiel make great ones) and add some soy cheese. Put the finished tofu scramble inside, wrap it up, and throw it in the oven for 15 minutes. Remove, plate, and top with some yogurt and chutney if you have it on hand. It's *dope!*

WAFFLES OR PANCAKES WITH FRESH MIXED BERRY COMPOTE

Makes 4–6 servings

If you don't have a waffle iron, just make pancakes with this batter. If you've got time, shut up the meatheads who say "What do you eat for breakfast, granola?" by making these with a side of the tofu scramble (page 194).

WAFFLES:

2½ cups organic flour
1 tbsp aluminum-free baking powder
1 tsp salt
1 tsp cinnamon
2 cups soy milk

1 cup sunflower oil

4 tsp Ener-G Egg Replacer

8 tbsp water

Earth Balance butter substitute

Organic maple syrup (nonorganic uses bad chemicals;
also, buy in bulk to get a better deal)

MIXED BERRY COMPOTE:

2 cups mixed berries (Whole Foods has an inexpensive
frozen mix)

⅓ cup agave syrup

¼ cup water

To make the waffles, begin by preheating your waffle
iron. Sift flour, baking powder, salt, and cinnamon together in a large bowl. Stir soy milk and oil into flour
mixture. In separate bowl, beat Egg Replacer with a
little water until foamy (about 30 seconds). Fold the dry
ingredients into Egg Replacer mixture. Cover and let sit
while you prepare the compote.

To make the compote, place berries, agave syrup (or
sugar), and water in a small saucepan over a very low
flame. Allow the berries to cook down to a thick, juicy
consistency (approx. 20 minutes). Remove from flame
and set aside.

Coat your heated waffle iron with a little Earth Balance spread. Pour a dollop of batter in the center of the iron and spread it out with a spatula until all of the squares are covered. Cook until edges turn golden brown and waffles fall off the iron without sticking. Melt some Earth Balance on each one, spoon some fresh fruit compote over the top, and add maple syrup.

LUNCH AND DINNER IDEAS

Most people work during the day, so I've included recipes here that are easy to bring to the office or job site. If you have kids, invite them into the kitchen and get them involved in learning about and preparing food. Most of these recipes are kid-friendly and can easily be packed up in lunch boxes.

VEGGIE CHILI WITH CORN BREAD

This chili is great on cold days and is loaded with nutrients. You can even fold in some chopped spinach or kale for an extra nutrition boost (this is an easy way to "hide" greens, if you're a parent).

CHILI:

Serves 4–6

2 cups dried kidney beans, soaked overnight (you can
    use drained and rinsed canned beans if you're
    short on time)

8 cups water

1 cup seitan, cubed

1 cup vegan soy meat, chopped

3 cups crushed ripe tomatoes

3 tbsp coconut oil

3 bay leaves

1 cup green pepper, chopped

2 fresh green chili peppers, chopped fine

1 cup carrots, chopped

1 tsp basil

1½ tsp oregano

1½ tsp cumin seeds

½ tsp coriander powder

¼ tsp cayenne pepper

1 tsp hing

2 tsp sea salt

½ cup Tofutti Sour Supreme

Bring the beans to a boil in a 4-quart soup pot. Cover

and simmer on a low flame until they get soft (approx. 2 hours). Add soy meat, tomatoes, and bay leaves and simmer covered for another 30 minutes.

Now the secret to a good chili: spicing. Heat the oil in a 12-inch frying pan and sauté seitan, green peppers, carrots, chili peppers, basil, hing, oregano, cumin, coriander, and chili powder until the seitan is evenly browned. Add this mixture to beans and throw in the salt and cayenne.

Place the Tofutti Sour Supreme on top of each serving. Serve with corn bread.

CORN BREAD:

Serves 8

Earth Balance Spread or canola oil, for greasing the pan
1 cup cornmeal
½ cup whole wheat pastry flour
½ cup unbleached white flour
2 tsp baking powder
1 cup soy milk
¼ cup olive oil
¼ cup maple syrup
½ tsp sea salt
½ cup grilled green and red bell peppers (optional)

Preheat oven to 350° F. Grease a 10-inch oven-safe round glass dish or a cast-iron baking dish with Earth Balance or oil. Get two bowls. In the first, mix together the cornmeal, whole wheat flour, white flour, and baking powder. In the second, whisk together soy milk, olive oil, maple syrup, and sea salt. Add the wet ingredients to the dry and stir in the grilled peppers if you chose to include them. Don't overmix, studly.

Pour this into your oiled baking dish and bake for approx. 25 minutes. Set aside to cool. Cut into wedges and serve with your chili. Or you can do some real Tex-Mex business and throw the bread in a dry frying pan until golden brown on each side.

GREEN SALAD WITH VINAIGRETTE

This is a very simple salad to make and the addition of raw beets and red cabbage makes it nutrient rich. Always remember to wash produce (even organic!) very well and dry the lettuce and spinach in a salad spinner.

Serves 4–6

2 heads of romaine lettuce
1 cup spinach, chopped
1 small beet, shredded

2 carrots, shredded

1 cup fresh red cabbage, shredded

2 cups sunflower sprouts

⅓ cup fresh walnuts

⅓ cup roasted pumpkin seeds

⅓ cup nori strips (super protein and iron)

Combine ingredients in a large bowl. Pour in dressing and toss to coat.

DRESSING:

½ cup apple cider

¼ cup rice vinegar

2 tbsp mirin

2 tbsp Nama Shoyu (amazing organic soy sauce)

1 tbsp olive oil

Combine all ingredients into a small bowl and whisk until oil and vinegar have emulsified.

BARBECUED TOFU

Makes 4 servings

Be prepared to look at tofu in a whole new light. I serve
this dish with mashed potatoes or yams, steamed collard
greens, corn on the cob, Earth Balance butter substitute,
and a splash of Bragg Liquid Aminos. You can even make
a tofu sandwich for work the next day. I like to add in
avocado and lettuce.

1 lb. extra-firm tofu
2 tbsp coconut oil
1 tsp hing
2 cloves garlic, peeled and chopped fine
¼ tsp hot pepper, seeded and crushed
¼ tsp thyme
pinch of garam masala
¼ tsp turmeric
½ tsp ginger, peeled and grated
½ tsp salt
¼ cup agave syrup
½ cup water
¼ cup pineapple juice
1 tbsp fresh lemon juice
1 tbsp organic brown mustard
pinch of Jamaican allspice

Preheat oven to 350° F. Slice the tofu into ¼-inch slices.
In a large saucepan, lightly fry in 1 tablespoon of oil and

set aside. Heat the remaining oil and sauté the garlic and hot pepper over a medium-low flame for one minute. Add all the remaining ingredients and simmer until the sauce reaches a smooth consistency, stirring frequently. Remove from heat and set aside.

Next, arrange your tofu slices on a nonstick baking sheet or dish and spread the sauce over the top of the tofu, making sure it's evenly covered. Bake for 15–20 minutes.

WHITE BEAN RICOTTA PASTA
by Rip Esselstyn

Makes 4 servings

Here's a great one from my homeboy, badass Rip Esselstyn, former firefighter/triathlete and author of the bestselling *Engine 2 Diet*. It's a delicious, healthy swap for traditional dairy-and-meat-heavy lasagna that would normally leave you in a coma after eating.

    16 oz whole grain ziti
    1 15-oz can white beans
    3 tbsp crushed garlic

3 tbsp Italian spice blend

½ cup frozen spinach (thawed)

2 tbsp nutritional yeast

1 jar tomato sauce

Preheat oven to 350° F.

Cook pasta according to instructions on box.

In a food processor, pulse all ingredients until smooth: white beans, garlic, spices, frozen spinach, and tomato sauce.

In a baking dish, create 1 layer of tomato sauce.

In a bowl, put in the rest of the tomato sauce and whole-grain pasta, and mix together.

Place in a baking pan on top of tomato sauce, and bake for 35 minutes.

Top with nutritional yeast.

TERIYAKI CHICK-N BURRITO WITH BASMATI RICE

Makes 4-6 servings

This is a hell of a decadent lunch. Use the basmati rice recipe below. Serve with steamed veggies. You can even add in some veggie chili to give your burrito a tasty, super-protein boost.

1 package of Gardein Teriyaki Chick-n strips
2 tbsp coconut oil
1 tsp fresh, finely grated ginger (skin removed)
2 cups Daiya cheese (optional)
1 cup nondairy, non-GMO sour cream
2 ripe avocados, sliced
2 cups spinach, washed and chopped fine
2 medium tomatoes, chopped
½ cup red bell peppers, chopped into small pieces
½ cup green bell peppers, chopped into small pieces
whole wheat tortillas (Rudi's are great)

Preheat oven to 400° F. Heat oil and then add ginger to the pan. After 30 seconds, drop in teriyaki strips. Brown on all sides and cook for approximately 5 minutes over medium flame. Add bell peppers and cook for 2 minutes until slightly tender. Add in glazing sauce (provided by Gardein). Stir strips and peppers, letting sauce coat them evenly. After 3 minutes, remove and set aside.

Lay tortillas on a flat surface and spread on sour cream. Add some of the strips/peppers combo, along with rice, grated cheese, and spinach. Roll and fold in the ends. Seal the edge with some sour cream. Place burritos in an oiled pan and cook in oven until tortillas turn golden brown (approx. 30 minutes). Remove and serve with your tomato and avocado.

BASMATI RICE

Makes 4–6 servings

Basmati rice is often used in Indian cooking and has a great nutty flavor. You can use red, brown, or white basmati; they all taste great. Here's my favorite recipe.

2 cups uncooked basmati rice
3½ cups water
1 tsp turmeric
1 tsp fresh, grated ginger (skin removed)
1 tsp cumin seeds
⅓ cup roasted cashews or pistachios
4 oz frozen peas
½ tsp black mustard seeds
2 tbsp Earth Balance butter substitute or coconut oil
2 tsp sea salt

Wash the rice and let it soak for 15 minutes. Then let it drain for 15 minutes. Put the water, salt, and frozen peas in a pot on high heat and bring to a boil. Heat the Earth Balance (or oil) in a medium-sized saucepan and fry the cumin and mustard seeds on medium heat.

When cumin seeds brown and mustard seeds pop, add the ginger and turmeric. Stir your spices together for 30 seconds so it becomes an even mixture. Add the rice and continue stirring for 2 minutes so all the spices and rice are mixed well and lightly toasted. Pour boiling water into the rice and add the nuts. Stir once, then cover and turn the heat to very low. Do not lift the lid. Cook until the rice has absorbed all the water (approx. 18–20 minutes).

IRONMAN STEW

Makes 6 servings

This is a hearty, flavorful veggie stew that's loaded with protein, vitamins, and minerals. It's great over brown rice or with salad, corn bread, or a thick-crusted bread like sourdough. Hint: it's even better the second day, when all the spices have soaked in.

5 tbsp coconut oil
2 cups potatoes, cubed and peeled
1½ cups mixed green and yellow zucchini
1½ cups carrots, sliced
2 cups green beans, chopped
2 cups broccoli florets
1 cup kale, chopped

1 cup spinach, chopped

2 cups mixed red and yellow cabbage

1 cup navy beans, soaked until tender

4 cups water

1 block extra-firm tofu, cut into 1-inch cubes

1½ cups Gardein Beefless Tips

2 tbsp tamari

1½ tsp dried thyme

2 tsp paprika

1 tsp dried basil

1 tsp ground cumin

1½ tsp hing

1½ tsp sea salt

½ tsp cayenne pepper

4 tbsp whole wheat flour

Grab a 4-quart soup pot and heat three tablespoons of the oil. Sauté the potatoes, carrots, and thyme. Once they get slightly tender, add all your veggies. Once everything is tender, throw in your navy beans and water. Simmer with the lid on and stir occasionally.

While that's all simmering, take a 10-inch frying pan and heat the rest of the oil. When it gets hot, add your tofu and Beefless Tips and sauté on a medium-low flame. Brown on all sides and pour in 1 tablespoon of tamari. Keep sautéing for 2 minutes and stir carefully so nothing burns or breaks. Now add this to your vegetables along with the rest of your tamari, spices, and salt.

Next drop the flour into a frying pan and brown it on a low flame. Do not let it burn. Take some of the water from your pot and slowly add it so it forms a paste. Make sure you get the lumps out. Add it to your soup pot once it becomes a bubbly mixture. Simmer this until all the veggies are tender and the beans are thoroughly cooked. Use a fork to test, not your teeth. If you cut through a bean and it's starchy and dry inside, cook a little while longer.

BEEFLESS SOFT TACOS WITH GREEN SALSA MARINADE AND AVOCADO SALSA
by Chef Tal Ronnen

Makes 3–6 servings

This recipe is from my boy, world-renowned chef Tal Ronnen. His book, *The Conscience Cook*, was a *New York Times* bestseller. He currently owns and operates Los Angeles's best gourmet veg restaurant, Crossroads. Tacos are fun to make; get the kids involved if you got 'em. Serve with a nice, big green salad.

1 bag Gardein Beefless Tips

6 small tortillas

1 cup prepared green salsa

2 tbsp chopped fresh cilantro

4 tbsp fresh lime juice

1½ tsp minced garlic

pinch sea salt

pinch black pepper

1 tbsp vegetable oil

½ avocado, diced

1 tbsp chopped onion

1 cup cooked corn

1 shredded green cabbage or romaine lettuce

BEEFLESS TIPS:

Defrost Beefless Tips for 5–10 minutes.

In a small bowl, make the marinade: Combine ⅓ cup of the prepared green salsa, 1 tbsp of the chopped cilantro, 2 tsp of the fresh lime juice, 1 tsp of the minced garlic, and salt and pepper to taste. Whisk together with a fork.

Cut Beefless Tips in half and place in shallow pan or roasting dish. Pour marinade over and allow to marinate for 20 minutes.

Heat stainless steel sauté pan, add oil, and sear Beefless Tips for 3 minutes on each side.

Meanwhile combine avocado salsa ingredients in medium bowl and set aside.

AVOCADO SALSA:

In a small bowl, combine the avocado and chopped onion with ⅔ cup of the prepared green salsa, 1 tbsp of the chopped cilantro, 2 tsp of the lime juice, and ½ tsp of the minced garlic.

Warm tortillas. Put Beefless Tips in middle of tortilla with avocado salsa, lettuce, and corn, then fold.

Garnish with your choice of green onions, shredded cheese, chopped fresh cilantro, and lime wedges.

TOMATO BISQUE WITH CASHEW CREAM
by Chef Tal Ronnen

Makes 6 servings

This recipe is also from Tal Ronnen and it's a dairy-free version of a favorite soup a lot of us grew up with. Serve this with your favorite veggie burger or with my Barbecued Tofu Sandwich (see page 202).

4 tbsp Earth Balance butter substitute

1 onion, chopped

1 celery stalk, chopped

1 carrot, chopped

3 cloves garlic, smashed

2 tbsp flour

5 cups faux chicken stock (Better Than Bouillon brand)
    or vegetable stock

1 can (15 oz) fire-roasted tomatoes

1 can (15 oz) diced tomatoes

2 tbsp parsley, chopped (optional)

2 sprigs thyme, leaves only

1 bay leaf

1½ cups cashew cream (recipe follows)

Add the Earth Balance to a large stockpot over medium heat. Heat until melted, but be careful not to let it burn. Add the onions, celery, carrots, and garlic. Cook for 10 minutes, stirring frequently. Sprinkle the flour over the vegetables and continue cooking for 2 minutes, stirring constantly.

Add the stock, tomatoes with juice, parsley, thyme, and bay leaf. Bring to a boil, reduce heat, and simmer for 30 minutes. Add the cashew cream and continue to simmer for 10 minutes; be careful not to let it boil.

Remove the bay leaf and, working in batches, purée the soup in a blender. Be careful not to overfill the blender; hot liquids tend to erupt. I try to keep it to about half capacity. You could also use an immersion blender if you have one. Return soup to pot to heat and serve.

CASHEW CREAM:

2 cups whole cashews (not pieces, which tend to be
    dried out)
Cold, filtered water

Put the cashews in a bowl and add cold water to cover them. Cover the bowl and refrigerate overnight.

Drain the cashews and rinse under cold water. Place them in a blender with enough fresh cold water to cover them by 1 inch. Blend on high for several minutes until very smooth.

To make thick cashew cream, which some of the recipes in this book call for, simply reduce the amount of water when they are placed in the blender, so that the water just slightly covers the cashews.

ALMOND FLAXSEED BURGER

by Brendan Brazier

Makes 2 servings

Here's a healthy veg burger idea from Brendan Brazier. Brendan designs every recipe to help you "thrive" in your fitness goals. Throw one of these tasty burgers on a sprouted Ezekiel bun with lettuce, tomato, sprouts, avocado, and eggless mayo for an easy dinner after you get home from the gym.

2 cloves garlic
1 cup almonds
½ cup ground flaxseed
2 tbsp balsamic vinegar
2 tbsp coconut oil, hemp oil, or EFA Oil Blend
sea salt to taste

Put all ingredients into a food processor. Process until well blended.

Process less if you prefer a coarser texture. Form into 2 patties.

Serve raw or, if you prefer to cook them, lightly cover with coconut oil and bake at 300° F for 35 minutes. Alternatively, lightly fry over medium until golden brown, flipping once.

SHAVED FENNEL SALAD WITH MANDARIN VINAIGRETTE
by Chef Chad Serno

Serves 4

These next two recipes are from my good friend and amazing chef Chad Sarno. Chad's been at this a long time and I consider him one of the world's best gourmet plant-based chefs. Check more of his recipes or get inspiration on his website (www.chadsarno .com)!

FENNEL AND FRUITS

2–3 fennel bulbs (2 cups), sliced paper thin, preferably using a mandolin
1 cup fresh sunflower sprouts
1 cup baby arugula
drizzle of mandarin vinaigrette (see recipe)

2 pears or apples, sliced paper thin, preferably using a
    mandolin
½ cup candied or toasted pecans, coarsely chopped

In small bowl, gently toss the shaved fennel,
sprouts, and arugula. Drizzle with mandarin vinaigrette, and top with a few slices of shaved pear
or apple. Sprinkle with toasted pecans and serve
immediately.

MANDARIN VINAIGRETTE

½ cup white wine or champagne vinegar
2 tbsp agave or sweetener of choice
¼ cup mandarin or orange segments, diced
2 tbsp finely chopped chives
2 tbsp finely chopped mint
1 tbsp orange zest
ground black pepper
pinch of sea salt

In small mixing bowl, combine all ingredients and whisk
together well.

JACKFRUIT CARNITA TACOS WITH AVOCADO AND PICKLED VEGETABLES

Jackfruit is the intimidating, massive fruit you have probably seen at your local Asian grocery store. It's one of the largest fruits on the planet and can reach up to fifty pounds! When you work with the unripe fruit, it has a very stringy texture, similar to shredded carnitas (pork). I made several batches of this to test it out, and was very happy with the results. The jackfruit carnitas were born!

You can buy jackfruit canned—be sure to get one with a saltwater brine (there are many varieties and some have funky ingredients). Or if you prefer you can substitute cubed tofu (1½ blocks), cubed tempeh (1½ packs), chopped hearts of palm, or artichoke hearts in place of the jackfruit.

Serves 6

2 cans green jackfruit, rinsed well, and core removed
2 tbsp olive oil
1 medium onion, diced
1 cup vegetable stock
1½ tsp oregano, fresh minced
¼ cup orange juice
juice of 1 lime

1 chipotle chili, in adobo sauce, minced

½ tsp chili powder

½ tsp onion granules

¼ tsp coriander powder

¼ tsp cinnamon

3 cloves garlic, minced

2 bay leaves

½ tsp black pepper

sea salt to taste

SERVE WITH:

Corn tortillas

avocado

pickled jalapeños and carrots (recipe follows)

your favorite salsa

Strain and rinse the jackfruit well. Place in mixing bowl.

Add the chipotle, chili, onion powder, coriander, cinnamon, garlic, and black pepper on the jackfruit, and shred pieces roughly while mixing. I prefer to allow this to sit and absorb the spices for at least an hour to overnight before cooking.

Place a small Dutch oven or shallow pot over medium heat. Add oil and diced onions and continuously stir until onions begin to brown. Add in remaining ingredients, including the spiced raw jackfruit.

Bring mixture to a simmer, breaking up the jackfruit by using a potato masher or a fork. Reduce heat to medium-low and cover.

Cook for 20 minutes, opening lid frequently to stir and break up larger pieces of jackfruit, ensuring it does not burn. Cook until all liquid has evaporated and the jackfruit begins to stick to pan. This is the sign that it's done.

Place a scoop of cooked jackfruit on a tortilla, and top with avocado, salsa, pickled jalapeños and carrots (recipe below), and cilantro.

PICKLED JALAPEÑOS AND CARROTS

6 jalapeños, sliced in thin rounds on mandolin

4 carrots sliced in thin rounds at an angle on mandolin

2 tbsp cilantro, chopped

1½ cups apple cider vinegar

½ tsp coriander seeds

4 garlic cloves, sliced thin

3 tbsp apricot paste

1 tsp sea salt

Place jalapeños, carrots, and cilantro in a medium-sized glass bowl.

In small saucepan over high heat, add the vinegar, coriander seeds, garlic, apricot paste, and sea salt and bring to a boil, whisking well. Remove from heat and pour over the veggies.

Allow to sit for at least an hour before using.

Pickled vegetables can be stored in an airtight container in the refrigerator for at least a week.

CITRUS "CHICKEN" AND VEGGIE STIR FRY

Makes 4 servings

Stir-frying is a plant-based eater's best friend. It's a quick and easy way to cook veggies and the results are so satisfying. I like to serve this gingery-citrusy stir fry over sticky coconut rice. It's the bomb!

> 1 14-oz Gardein Mandarin Orange Crispy Chik'n
> 3 tbsp tamari (a thick soy sauce)
> 4 tbsp arrowroot powder
> 3 tbsp apple cider
> 2 tbsp fresh lemon juice
> pinch of cayenne
> 2 tbsp coconut oil
> 2 cups broccoli, chopped
> 2 tbsp ginger, peeled and minced

1 cup bok choy, sliced
½ cup red bell peppers, sliced in long strips
½ cup yellow squash, sliced in one-inch strips

Prepare Gardein according to the recipe on the box and set aside.

Then make your sauce. Mix the arrowroot in ½ cup water and heat in a small saucepan over low flame. Once it thickens, remove from heat and stir in the tamari, lemon juice, cider, and cayenne. Cover and set aside.

Heat the oil in a skillet over medium flame. Sauté the broccoli and ginger for 3 minutes. Stir in all your veggies and Gardein strips. Cook until all the veggies are tender. Remove from flame and stir in sauce, tossing to coat. Serve with rice or your grain of choice.

COCONUT RICE

Makes 4 servings

2 cups organic jasmine rice
2 cups coconut milk
1¾ cups water
½ tsp salt

½ tsp coconut oil

1 tsp organic unprocessed sugar

2 tbsp toasted coconut flakes for garnish

Rub the oil over the bottom of a medium-sized pot. Place rice, coconut milk, water, and salt in the pot and bring to a simmer over medium-high heat. Stir well. Add the sugar. Continue to stir occasionally until the coconut milk and water come to a gentle boil. Turn the heat down to medium-low and place the lid slightly askew on the pot so steam can escape. Cook until the rice has absorbed all the coconut-water mix (15–20 minutes).

Now turn off the heat, but leave the pot on the burner. Cover the pot tightly with the lid and allow it to sit for 5–10 minutes or until you're ready to eat. The rice will steam and have a nice, slightly sticky texture. Garnish with the toasted coconut flakes.

CHICKPEA AND LENTIL BALLS WITH TAHINI SAUCE
by Chef Jorge Pineda

Makes 4–6 servings

Jorge is one of the chefs at New York's plant-based gourmet restaurant, Candle 79. I am so honored to call owners Joy

Pierson and Bart Potenza my friends. I know of no restaurant owners in the city who do more to help the underprivileged and needy gain access to healthy organic food that tastes out-of-this-world amazing. They are also part of the team involved in the Healthy School Lunch Program in New York and work endlessly to help others. We need millions like those two!

LENTIL AND CHICKPEA BALLS:

3 cups cooked chickpeas (about 1 cup uncooked)
1 cup beluga lentils, cooked
⅓ cup chopped celery
⅓ cup chopped onions
4 tbsp extra-virgin olive oil
1 tsp sea salt
1 tsp cumin
1 tbsp smoked paprika
2 tbsp chopped parsley
¼ cup unbleached flour

TAHINI SAUCE:

¼ cup tahini
¼ cup water
2 tbsp lemon juice
2 tbsp parsley

2 tsp mirin

1 tsp toasted sesame oil

1 tsp agave nectar

1 tsp tamari

Place the chickpeas in a bowl and cover with water. Let them soak overnight. Drain the water from the chickpeas and put in a medium pot with enough water to cover the chickpeas by an inch. Bring to a boil and then reduce heat and simmer for 45–50 minutes or until the chickpeas are tender. When chickpeas are cooked, drain the liquid and allow to cool. In a large pot, bring 4 cups of water to a boil and add the lentils and the salt. Simmer 20–25 minutes over medium-high heat. Drain the liquid and allow the lentils to cool. In a large sauté pan over medium heat, sauté the onions and celery in extra-virgin olive oil and let cool.

Preheat oven to 350° F. Put the chickpeas in a food processor for 5 minutes or until ground. Combine all ingredients in bowl and mix together. Form mixture into 2-inch balls and place on a greased baking sheet. Put in the oven and bake for 15 minutes or until golden brown.

To make tahini sauce, place all the sauce ingredients in a blender and blend for 1–2 minutes or until smooth. To serve put 3–4 balls in a pita bread with chopped lettuce, tomato, and red onion, and drizzle with tahini sauce.

COCONUT MINT CURRY
by Chef Darshana Thacker

Makes 4 servings

This recipe is from my good friend Darshana Thacker. Darshana is a plant-based chef who is well known in the yoga community of Los Angeles. She specializes in contemporary interpretations of the traditional cooking she learned in her mother's kitchen growing up in India.

> 1 medium or ½ cup red onion, cut into big pieces
> 2 cloves garlic
> 1½-inch piece or 1½ tbsp ginger, grated
> 1 cup water
> 1½ cup green beans, cut into ½-inch pieces
> 1 cup carrots, cut into small pieces
> 1 cup zucchini, cut into small pieces
> 1½ cup cauliflower, cut into small florets
> 1 cup coconut milk
> ½ tsp salt or to taste
> ½ tsp garam masala
> ½ tsp turmeric
> 2 tsp curry powder (mild)

1 tsp lime juice
¼ cup cilantro, finely chopped
¼ cup fresh mint, finely chopped

To a blender, add the onion, garlic, ginger, and ½ cup water and blend until smooth.

Pour onion mixture into a shallow pan, cover, and cook on medium-low heat for 10 minutes. Add the green beans and ½ cup water; continue to cook covered for 7–8 minutes. Add the carrots and cook for another 5 minutes, or until carrots are soft.

Add the cauliflower, zucchini, coconut milk, salt, garam masala, turmeric, and curry powder. Cover and cook for 10–15 minutes. Uncover and stir in the lime juice, mint, and cilantro. Serve hot with rice.

SWEET-AND-SOUR TOFU BALLS OVER QUINOA

Makes 4 servings

Yeah, it's fried . . . so shoot me in the fucking head. Listen, people—a fried dish every now and then won't kill ya. Loosen up and enjoy a little!

TOFU BALLS:

2 cups firm organic tofu (or at least non-GMO tofu)
2 tbsp whole wheat flour
½ tsp salt
1 cup fresh pineapple with juice, chopped (use canned
    if necessary, just not with white sugar syrup)
5 tbsp apple cider vinegar
3 tbsp raw organic sugar
2 tbsp tamari
1 tbsp cornstarch, blended in ⅓ cup pineapple juice
¾ cup safflower oil for deep frying

Drain all the water out of the tofu by squeezing it. Place tofu in a bowl and mash well with the back of a spoon, draining any excess water that is released. Stir in salt and flour until combined. Form tofu into small balls.

In a shallow (12-inch) pan heat oil until shimmering over medium-high heat. Do not let oil smoke—if the oil begins to smoke, you have overheated it and you need to discard it and begin again. Carefully add the tofu to the oil and deep-fry in the oil until golden brown. Place cooked tofu on paper-towel-lined plate to drain.

In a large saucepan over medium-high heat, place apple cider vinegar, sugar, tamari, and cornstarch mixture. Bring to a boil and stir gently until the mixture thickens. Add the tofu balls and pineapple. Simmer for 3–4 minutes.

QUINOA:

2 cups water
½ cup cashew pieces
½ tsp salt
pinch turmeric
1 cup quinoa

In a medium saucepan, bring water, cashews, salt, and turmeric to a boil. Add quinoa, then stir and lower flame. Simmer covered for 10–15 minutes until water is evaporated and quinoa is fluffy.

VEGGIE CHICKEN AND RICE CASSEROLE

Makes 4 servings

This dish is rich and sticks to your ribs. I've converted many a Neanderthal meat-eater to the veggie side with this one. Enjoy!

2 tbsp sesame oil
2 cups non-GMO seitan veggie chicken sliced into thin
    1-inch strips
2 tbsp nutritional yeast
1½ cups Daiya cheddar cheese, grated

½ cup Daiya Italian blend cheese, grated

¼ cup cold-pressed olive oil

1 tsp black mustard seeds

½ tsp cumin powder

½ tsp hing

½ tsp turmeric

3 tomatoes

1 bunch of spinach, washed and stemmed

4 cups cooked basmati rice

1½ cups broccoli florets, steamed

1 carrot, chopped and steamed

1 tsp salt

¼ tsp black pepper

¼ cup whole wheat bread crumbs

Preheat oven to 350° F.

In a medium-sized pan, heat the oil over medium-high heat. Add veggie chicken strips and sear, turning once, so they're crispy on all sides but still tender (4–5 minutes). Remove strips from pan and set aside.

In a bowl, lightly toss yeast with the grated cheeses so it sticks together.

Heat the olive oil in a 12-inch frying pan over medium heat and add mustard seeds. When they crackle, add cumin, hing, turmeric, and tomatoes. Sauté for 5 minutes, stirring occasionally so tomatoes pick up the spices. Add spinach and sauté 3 more minutes.

In a large bowl, combine the rice, veggie strips, and steamed and sautéed veggies. Stir in the salt and pepper and bread crumbs. Top with cheese mixture, reserving a little. Stir to just combine, but don't overmix ingredients.

Put everything in a 2-quart casserole dish and sprinkle the remaining cheese. Cover and bake for 15 minutes. Remove cover and bake 10 minutes more.

SPAGHETTI WITH VEGGIE NO-MEATBALLS

Makes 4 servings

This dish rocks! I like to serve it with some greens—a simple green salad or steamed broccoli, kale, or spinach. Whole Foods and most Indian grocery stores will have all the spices you need. If you make a salad, avoid using iceberg lettuce; opt for dark green leafy romaine, which is higher in chlorophyll.

1 pound organic whole wheat pasta (cook as directed)

SAUCE:
¼ cup olive oil
2 tbsp coconut oil
½ tsp black mustard seeds

1 small, fresh green chili, chopped fine

2 tsp fresh basil, chopped

2 tsp salt

½ tsp asafetida

½ tsp cumin powder

1 tsp black pepper

6 plum tomatoes, chopped into eighths

2 jars organic tomato sauce

2 tsp organic blackstrap molasses

To make the sauce, heat oils in medium-sized pan over medium heat. Add mustard seeds and fry for 45 seconds or until they begin to pop. Add your chili, basil, and powdered spices. Cook for one minute and add chopped tomatoes. Cook tomatoes for 5 minutes, stirring, until they have reduced to a thick paste. Then add sauce and bring to a boil. Add molasses and reduce to simmer for 30 minutes. Cover and keep warm.

VEGGIE NO-MEATBALLS:

2 cups grated cauliflower

2 cups grated cabbage

1½ cups garbanzo bean flour

½ cup Daiya mozzarella

1½ tsp salt

1 tsp ground cumin

½ tsp hing

1 tsp garam masala

½ tsp coriander powder

½ tsp turmeric

pinch of cayenne

¾ cup oil for deep frying (sunflower or something else light)

Combine all veggie meatball ingredients in a bowl. The moisture from the cauliflower and cabbage will make it thick; you don't need to add water. Form into 24 balls about an inch in diameter each.

Heat oil in a medium-sized saucepan until it is very hot. Don't let the oil begin to smoke; if it does, discard oil and start again. Test your oil by dropping in a small piece of meatball. If it floats to the top and cooks, you're ready. Working in batches, fry until golden brown. Remove cooked meatballs and place on paper-towel-lined plate to drain.

Add meatballs to the warm sauce and let them soak for one hour. Cook pasta according to package directions. Serve sauce and meatballs over pasta and sprinkle with Daiya cheese.

Here's another idea. Make some extra balls and leave soaking in the sauce overnight. Heat the next day and make a no-meatball sub with soy cheese. If you have a George Foreman Grill (I do, but no meat has ever touched it) or a panini press, use it so the bread gets toasted and crunchy. Or you can just wrap in foil and place in a preheated oven at 450° for twenty minutes. It's off the chart, fellas.

SOBA SENSATION SAUCE WITH STEAMED VEGGIES, QUINOA, AND BLACK BEANS

Makes 3 cups

This quick, amazing recipe is from my good friend the beautiful Leslie McEachern, who is the owner of Angelica Kitchen on East Twelfth Street in New York. She's been open since 1976 and has a cult following—I'm one of her many disciples. When I was living in burnt-out buildings on the Lower East Side in 1980, she would feed all of us every night, giving us the leftovers from the restaurant. She was a huge facilitator in my going plant based. I'm still at the restaurant all the time and she still warms the place with her wonderful spirit. She embodies the true meaning of philanthropy. Okay . . . now on to her incredible food.

SOBA SENSATION SAUCE:

1 clove garlic, crushed
3 tbsp minced fresh ginger
2 tbsp Dijon mustard
⅓ cup rice vinegar (not sweetened)
⅓ cup tamari sauce
⅓ cup light rice syrup
2 tbsp toasted sesame oil
1⅓ cups tahini (sesame seed paste)
⅓ cup hot water
pinch of cayenne pepper

Combine all ingredients with hot water in a blender or food processor and blend until smooth. Thin the sauce with more water if you choose.

Serve over steamed kale, carrots, and squash along with quinoa and black beans for a very healthy quick meal.

ROASTED VEGETABLE MEDLEY FOR GRAINS, BEANS, OR BAKED POTATOES

Makes 6–8 servings

Here is a great recipe from my homeboy and amazing chef Mike Perrine.

You can enhance any grain or bean dish by folding in these vegetables. I also like to spoon this veggie medley over baked potatoes.

2 cups diced peppers
2 cups diced zucchini
2 cups chopped cauliflower (blanched for 1 minute)
½ cup diced fennel or celery
1 tsp Celtic sea salt
2 cups diced asparagus

DRESSING FOR VEGETABLES:

2 tbsp extra-virgin olive oil
½ tsp dry oregano
½ tsp dry basil
1 tsp hing
¼ tsp Celtic sea salt
1 tbsp fresh thyme, rosemary, or sage
fresh ground pepper to taste

On a parchment-lined baking sheet spread the diced peppers, zucchini, and blanched cauliflower.

Place into a 375° F oven for 30 minutes. Remove sheet from oven and stir the vegetables around to ensure they cook evenly. Place it back in the oven and bake for another 20 minutes. Stir again and finish with 5 more minutes in the oven, then remove and cool.

Add the celery, carrots, and sea salt to a sauté pan. Sweat out the celery on medium heat until soft. Add a splash of water if necessary.

Blanch the asparagus for 45 seconds in salted boiling water. Remove and cool.

When cooled to room temperature or slightly warmer, combine all of the vegetables with the oil and herbs and serve over beans, grains, or sweet potatoes.

HEALTHY GREEN BEANS ALMONDINE

Makes 4 servings

This is great as a side dish to any entrée—it is always a hit at my place. Unlike those gross green bean casseroles you may have grown up with, this version is healthy and way more delicious thanks to a nice dose of spice.

1½ pounds fresh string beans

1 cup spinach, washed, stemmed, and chopped

3 tbsp coconut oil

2 tbsp shredded (fine) coconut

¼ tsp hing

1 tsp salt

¼ tsp black pepper

1 tsp ground coriander

½ cup slivered almonds

Snip off the ends of the beans and slice them into thin strips. Heat oil in a heavy cast-iron skillet and add hing, stirring, until fragrant. Add beans, pepper, salt, and 2 tablespoons of water. Cover and cook over medium heat until beans are tender, 10–15 minutes. Remove cover and cook for an additional 5 minutes. When the water has evaporated add almonds, shredded coconut, and spinach and cook for 5 minutes longer. Add coriander and serve hot. If you want a buttery flavor, you can add a teaspoon of Earth Balance.

RICE WITH DAL AND CHAPATI

This is a traditional Indian dish that is super-tasty. You can eat this any way you prefer, but I like to pour a bit of dal (soup) over the rice on my plate, then use the chapati (flat bread) to wrap it up with some greens, like a little packet. Delicious.

Basmati Rice (recipe page 207)

DAL:

1 cup split mung beans, soaked in water for 1 hour, rinsed and drained

7 cups water

½ tsp turmeric

1 cup carrot, diced

2 cups small cauliflower florets or 2 cups small broccoli florets (or 1 cup each of cauliflower and broccoli florets)

3 tbsp Earth Balance

3 tbsp cumin seeds or 3 tbsp cumin, to meet your taste preferences

½ tsp fennel seed

1–2 chiles, seeded and chopped

1 tbsp fresh gingerroot, chopped

¼ cup fresh coriander leaves, chopped

3 tbsp fresh lemon juice

1 tsp salt

¼ tsp black pepper

Add the mung beans, water, turmeric, and carrots to a heavy-based medium pan over high heat and bring the water to the boil; reduce the heat and allow the contents of the pan to simmer, semi-covered, for 15 minutes, or until the mung beans start to break down. Add the cauliflower florets to the pan and simmer for another 10 minutes.

Meanwhile, heat the Earth Balance in a small pan over medium heat; add the cumin and fennel seeds and gently cook them, stirring occasionally, until they have darkened a few shades; add the chilies and ginger and continue cooking until aromatic.

Pour the contents of the pan into the simmering soup; stir in the fresh coriander leaves, lemon juice, salt, and pepper. Serve hot.

CHAPATI:

1 cup whole wheat flour
¼ cup melted Earth Balance (optional)
½ tsp sea salt
warm water

Mix the flour, water, and salt together, adding water gradually until dough is soft but not wet, and can be kneaded. Knead the dough until it's fairly soft (8–10 minutes). Cover and let dough rest for one hour. Sprinkle flour on rolling area and make 1½-inch balls out of dough. Flatten balls and roll out to about 4–5 inches in diameter. Place the chapati on a heated skillet (dry, free from oil) and cook until bubbles appear. Turn chapati quickly and let cook until bubbles appear again. Using tongs, remove chapati from pan, and hold over an open flame or burner to make it puff up. Heat it first on the side that was first cooked. You can lay it directly on the burner for a brief moment, but don't let it stick. When chapati puffs up, turn quickly and repeat on other side till it puffs. Remove and butter both sides, and then cover until all chapatis are finished.

SNACKS AND DESSERT

HUMMUS

This is another recipe courtesy of Leslie McEachern of NYC's Angelica Kitchen. Hands down it's some of the best hummus I've ever had. You can serve it with pita bread or get creative. Use the chapati recipe (page 240) and make wraps by adding lettuce, tomato, sprouts, and avocado with some egg-free mayo.

Makes 4 cups

1½ cups dried chickpeas
6 cups water and additional water
½ cup tahini
⅔ cup freshly squeezed lemon juice, strained
2 cloves garlic, halved lengthwise
1 tsp ground cumin
¾ tsp sea salt
pinch of cayenne pepper
¾ cup water (or reserved chickpea cooking liquid)

Soak the chickpeas for 8 hours in the 6 cups of water. Drain the chickpeas, place in a 2–3 quart saucepan, and cover with fresh water by 2 inches. Bring to a boil, lower the heat, cover, and simmer for 2–3 hours or until the chickpeas are tender. Drain and reserve cooking liquid.

Combine chickpeas, tahini, lemon juice, garlic, cumin, salt, and cayenne in a food processor fitted with a steel blade. With the machine running gradually, add cooking liquid, processing until the mixture is creamy and smooth. If the sides become caked with the bits of unpuréed chickpeas, scrape down the sides with a rubber spatula. Taste to adjust the seasonings. Serve with pita and black olives.

Notes: You can speed up the cooking time by placing the chickpeas in 2–3-quart pressure cooker, covering the chickpeas by 1 inch, cooking for 45 minutes. Also, if the chickpeas are taking too long to soften (while soaking), you can add a little baking powder to the water. If you want the chickpeas to hold their shape for a salad, don't pressure-cook for any longer than 30 minutes.

KALE CHIPS

Serves 3

Kale is rich in calcium, iron, vitamin A, vitamin C, and bone-building vitamin K. It contains seven times the beta-carotene of broccoli. Kale chips are such an easy way to get some nutrients into your day, and with this recipe you'll spend a fraction of what you would buying them—I've seen kale chips going for eight dollars a box at health food stores in New York.

If you don't have a dehydrator (yet) you can use your oven.

> 1 bunch fresh kale
> 2 tsp tahini
> 1 tsp raw apple cider vinegar
> 1 tsp tamari

½ tsp raw agave nectar
3 tbsp nutritional yeast
¼ tsp turmeric
pinch of paprika powder
pinch of cumin powder
pinch of hing
pinch of Himalayan sea salt

Line two baking sheets with parchment paper. Turn oven on to lowest temperature and preheat (mine starts at 100° F).

Meanwhile, wash the kale by submerging it in a bowl of cold water. Dirt tends to get in the creases of the leaves, so be thorough. Pull the leaves from the thick stems and dry them. I use a salad spinner. You have to get *all* the water off and make them as dry as possible.

In a large bowl, combine the tahini, vinegar, tamari, and agave nectar. Stir through until completely smooth. Add kale and toss, mixing with the tahini. Add the nutritional yeast, salt, and spices, and keep tossing. Place kale on the baking sheets and place in the oven.

Bake at 100–150° F for an hour, then rotate trays, letting them bake for another 40 minutes. Increase oven temperature to 170° F, and let bake for another 20 minutes.

If kale is dry and crispy, remove from oven. If not, turn off heat and let kale sit in the warmth until crispy. A dehydrator is much easier and the chips come out perfect, so I suggest you get one. Always store these in an airtight container; otherwise the chips will break apart and turn to dust.

VERY BERRY PEACH CRISP

Serves 8–10

I try to avoid sugar, so this fruit-based dessert satisfies my craving when I want something sweet. If peaches aren't in season, try using nectarines or pears. It is delicious à la mode with some coconut ice cream. Just make sure you train the next day!

    3 cups peaches, sliced thin
    1 cup fresh blueberries
    1 cup fresh blackberries
    1 cup fresh raspberries
    2 tbsp lemon juice
    1 cup Earth Balance butter substitute
    ½ cup apple juice
    3 tbsp maple syrup

¼ cup walnuts, chopped

¼ cup pecans, chopped

1 tsp vanilla flavor (*not* extract)

4 cups rolled oats

1½ cups whole wheat pastry flour

1 tsp allspice

½ tsp salt

Preheat oven to 375° F. Grease a 9x13 baking dish with Earth Balance.

Place peaches in a large bowl and pour the lemon juice over the top. Add berries and gently stir to combine. Set aside.

In a small saucepan, melt butter substitute over low heat. Add in apple juice and maple syrup. Remove from heat and let cool to room temperature.

In a large bowl, combine nuts, vanilla, oats, flour, allspice, and salt. Stir in butter mixture until well combined. Pour half of this mixture into a baking dish. Top with fruit, spreading evenly. Pour the remaining mixture over the fruit and bake for 35 minutes, or until golden brown on top. Let cool for one hour and serve warm.

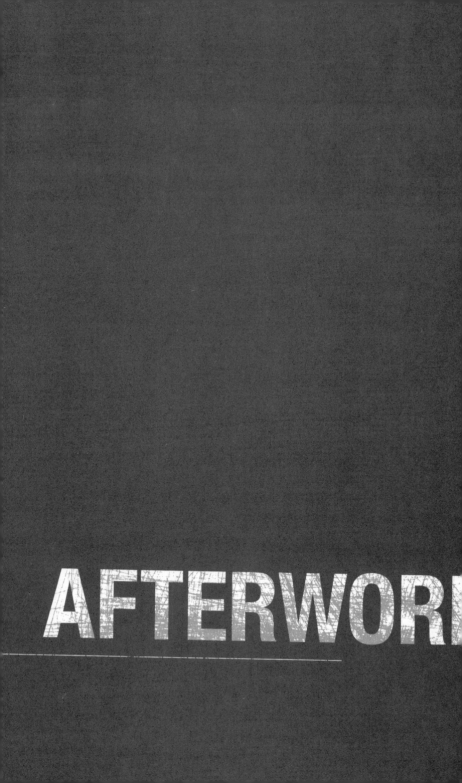

AFTERWORD

by Fred Bisci

John Joseph's in-your-face, kick-in-the-groin style of writing will definitely get your attention. As I went through his book, I got the impression that his early years were one big brawl through the dark side of life. Then John was fortunate enough to have an encounter with the truth. He realized he had to change. He went from slugging his way through life and living on the edge to a more peaceful life, free of animal flesh. His journey is pretty amazing, and I found John Joseph's book as attention getting as a left hook to the jaw.

John's book really hits home for me. I was born in October 1929, on the eve of the first big depression of the twentieth century, and I've experienced a good number of physical, emotional, and spiritual brawls in my eighty-four years of life. If you have the eyes to see, you'll observe people around you whose physical vitality is rapidly waning. Many of us are dangerously overweight. Obesity in this country is in epidemic proportions, which in many cases results in coronary artery disease, type 2 diabetes, and kidney and liver problems. The majority of times this is a result of processed foods, excessive animal protein, and the chemicals that are used in the processing and denaturing of these foods. My recommendation for people is to eliminate processed food and to live on an organic, whole-food, plant-based diet.

Our bodies have been poisoned by processed "foods" and our society is plagued by degenerative diseases that were rarities in previous generations. How many people do you know who are suffering from or have died from cancer or heart disease? What are your chances of escaping a similar fate? Some researchers predict that over the next ten years, 25 percent of all men will be diagnosed with prostate cancer. Yes, one out of every four men. Women don't fare any better, since the statistics for contracting breast cancer are of the same order of magnitude. And this is just one form of one disease. Do a calculation based on all types of cancer and heart disease, then add in the other common degenerative diseases, and you'll see why the future of our society looks bleak.

Worse still, it's not just our bodies that are degenerating. The mind, body, and spirit are all interdependent. So when one of them is in decline, so are the others, whether or not it's apparent on the surface. Therefore, our ailing bodies are a sure indicator that we're also in emotional and spiritual trouble. Look around you again and you'll see signs everywhere that this is so.

Fortunately, there's also some very good news: the remedy for this dreadful state of affairs is simple. Notice that I said simple, not easy. It's simple because it can be stated in a couple of sentences: stop consuming toxic foods that are not suited to the biochemical makeup of your body, and instead return to a *natural, healthy lifestyle* composed primarily of raw fruits, vegetables, nuts, seeds, and sprouts, the right whole grains, and legumes. Eat these foods in the correct combination and sequences, and avoid overeating.

In my forty-seven years of experience counseling thousands of people, the best results I have seen have come from a whole-food, plant-based diet. Doing this runs counter to ingrained habits, long-standing addictions, vested interests on the part of business, and our reluctance as a society to work for long-term goals rather than short-term. The processed food industry, pharmaceutical business, and many parts of the medical establishment do not want to see any changes in the standard American diet because this is a multibillion-dollar business.

As John Joseph has stated in his book, I've been slugging it out for forty-five years to open people's minds and hearts to simple truth. During that time I've studied nutritional science in great detail, gathered data by working with tens of thousands of clients, and above all used my own body as a living laboratory. What I've seen is the human body's effectiveness to demonstrate health time and time again if you allow it to. I'm not going to promise that you'll live to the age of 120 with no illnesses, though such an outcome is possible. What I can say is that even though genetic and environmental factors may limit what you can achieve, if you apply healthy lifestyle principles you will *live longer* and enjoy far *better health*—in mind, body, and spirit—than you will if you continue with your current routine.

At eighty-four years of age, looking back on my life I am quite sure that I would not have the quality of life I have now or might not even be here if I was not free of *all* animal products.

If you want to get healthy and help save this planet, you picked up the right book.

—*Fred Bisci, author of* Your Healthy Journey

ACKNOWLEDGMENTS

Special thanks to my creative director, Todd Irwin.

Srila Prabhupada, Radha/Govinda (protector of the cows), Brahma Bhuta, Vani Devi Dasi, my main man and member of the Trinity, without whom none of this would be possible. Dan Kirschen!; my incredible editor, Julie Will; and the most awesome Karen Rinaldi and Sydney Pierce at HarperWave. Mom, E, Frank Sr., Frank White (Superstar), Sean McGowan, Sandra S., Fred Bisci, Rory, Jen Irwin, AJ Novello, Mackie, Elle +1, the D'Angelo family, the Lastraglia family, Uncle John and Aunt Madeline, Chloe Jo Berman and Jeremy, David, Ivan and the DC3 Crew—Kap, Yama, Melissa, and our first editor, Josh Riman, Rory Freedman, Mike Perrine, Ravi, Tal Ronnen,

Iliya (Bonobos), Mac Danzig, Ray Lego, Rich Roll, Rip Esselstyn, Brendan Brazier, Jake Shields, Mike Mahler, Mark, Ali, Mike Dijon, Chris Garver, Doug Mackinnon, Artie McGuck (wtf), Shaun Fowler, Orion Mims, Ian Norrington, Aaron Drogoszewski, Erika Mitchener, Ajay James, Brian Wendel, Dr. Robert Ostfeld, Dave Navarro, Todd Newman, Anthony Baugh, Cherrie Laygo, Stephanie Swane, Nancy Friedman, Bojana, Sabrina, Danny Ilchuk, Davey AFI, Toby, Moon and Max (super-veg fam), Boogie, Karuna, Clayton Patterson, Lars and Tim (Rancid), Bryan and Vicki Callen, Jay Dublee (raw food Sadhu), Bad Brains, Moby, Benay, Bart and Joy (Candle 79), Tim Borer, Gretchen Ryan and fam, Dan (Montreal Crew), Randy (Lamb of God), Onno and fam, Beast, Darryl M. and the Detroit crew, Medium Al, Masha Rudenko, Francis B, Uncle Mike Schnapp, Steve Marcus, Nimai, Gee Bee, Keene, Louise (CBGB), Gene Stone, Guy Lesser, Al Barr (Dropkicks), Aaron, Doug Greene and the Liquiteria posse, Peter Nusbaum, Joe (Viva Herbal Pizzeria, NYC), Doug Crosby, Paul Haggis, Cindy Frey, Josh G (Clockwork Jiu Jitsu, NYC), Frank Grillo and fam, Jack and Jill Marshall, Joshua Katcher, Chris (DMS), Joe Hardcore, Chopper and fam, Trevor and fam, Vinnie (Generation Records), Christian (Zoo York), Craig Setari, Pete and S.O.I.A., Patty Jenkins, Sam Sheridan, Darius (Sid's Bike Shop, NYC), Eric (Bicycle Habitat, NYC), Melissa F, Paul

Kemawikasit, Saint Mark's Books, Ian McKae, PETA, Robert Cheeke, Dave Stein, Steve Martin (N.L.M.), Gene Baur (Farm Sanctuary), Pete Cervoni, Mike Da Monk, Alicia Silverstone, Bleu, Leslie and the Angelica's Crew, Jimmy G (future veg), Cousin Joe, Freddy Madball, David and Molly (Madeleine Bistro, Cali), and special thanks to all vegan and animal rights warriors worldwide who give a voice to the innocent, suffering earthlings. CUZ MEAT IS MURDER!!!

APPENDIX

Earth to Humans . . . Payback's a Bitch

Nothing will benefit human health and increase chances for survival of life on Earth as much as the evolution to a vegetarian diet.

—ALBERT EINSTEIN

It cracks me up when I see "environmentalist" celebrities support their cause by serving five-hundred-dollar Kobe beef steaks at their fund-raisers. Sure, they probably drove a hybrid electric car to their fancy dinner, but guess what? While not everyone on earth drives a car, everyone has to eat. Food therefore should be one of your biggest concerns if you give a shit about the planet we live on. Because a planet that needs to sustain a meat-based diet for its billions of inhabitants is a planet that will become sick.

Since the 1950s, the consumption of meat has almost doubled in this country. One reason is that the cost of buying meat has greatly decreased. Meat used to be a luxury that only rich people could afford (in fact, diseases like gout and obesity were considered upper-class illnesses). But today, you can buy a burger for ninety-nine cents. How did that happen?

The answer lies in how our meat is produced. Raising animals on small-scale family farms is costly. Raising animals on large-scale factory farms is cheap. It's also necessary to meet the world's ever-increasing meat demands. But this increase in meat consumption and production has not only impacted our health negatively— it has also impacted the planet in some pretty fucking horrible ways.

I've heard scumbags respond to this information by saying, "Man, fuck the future generations that have to pay for all the shit I'm doing to the planet because of my food choices. I live in the here and now. I'll have my steaks, rotisserie chicken, pork chops, eggs, and fish sticks, and I'll eat them too." Nice, douche bag. But guess what? Your "here and now" is turning into shit as well.

And then there are those who pay lip service to the idea of supporting the environment. The whole "Go Green" thing has become the catchphrase of the day—I've even seen it on the windows of fast-food hamburger joints.

In the middle of these extremes you have the crowd who thinks they aren't doing any harm to the environment because they only eat local, organic, free-range animals. Well, whooptie-fucking-doo, Prescott and Penelope, your cow may have been happy before it was slaughtered for your dinner, but the fact is you're still contributing to the destruction of the planet.

James McWilliams, author of *Just Food: Where Locavores Get It Wrong and How We Can Truly Eat Responsibly*, wrote about the environmental impact of the "grass-fed" movement in an op-ed piece for the *New York Times* in April 2012 and helped put this movement into perspective.[39] "It requires 2 to 20 acres to raise a cow on grass. If we raised all the cows in the United States on grass (all 100 million of them), cattle would require (using the figure of 10 acres per cow) almost half the country's land, and this figure excludes space needed for pastured chicken and pigs. A tract of land just larger than France has been carved out of the Brazilian rain forest and turned over to grazing cattle. Nothing about this is sustainable."

That's pretty spot-on, if you ask me. And by the way, free-range chickens and pigs are just as bad when you consider all the water and land required to maintain them, not to mention the vast amount of fossil fuels needed to produce the grains fed to those animals just so you can eat them.

The truth is, anyone who supports any aspect of these industries is contributing to the destruction of this planet. Five years ago, a report by the Pew Charitable Trusts and Johns Hopkins Bloomberg School of Public Health blasted the meat industry for the "unintended consequences" of factory farming practices: endangering public health, the environment, animal welfare, and rural communities. And in 2010, the United Nations urged a global shift away from meat and dairy, stating, "As the global population surges towards a predicted 9.1 billion people by 2050, Western tastes for diets rich in meat and dairy products are unsustainable."[40] The report, issued from the United Nations Environment Programme's International Panel of Sustainable Resource Management, went on to say, "Impacts from agriculture are expected to increase substantially due to population growth increasing consumption of animal products. Unlike fossil fuels, it is difficult to look for alternatives: people have to eat. A substantial reduction of impacts would only be possible with a substantial worldwide diet change, away from animal products."

842 million people in the world do not have enough to eat, and growing livestock for meat wastes an astronomical amount of land and water that could be used to feed people. We can produce far more vegetarian meals using the same amount of resources.

Here's a quick breakdown of how many people can be fed by the food produced on 2.5 acres of land, using various farming techniques.

Cabbage	23 people
Potatoes	22 people
Rice	19 people
Corn	17 people
Wheat	15 people
Chicken	2 people
Milk	2 people
Eggs	1 person
Beef	1 person

(Cited in *The Food Revolution* by John Robbins)

And as recently as 2013, the Johns Hopkins Center for a Livable Future also called out the meat industry for getting worse, not better. Hazards like liquid waste from huge animal operations, rampant and unnecessary use of antibiotics, inhumane treatment of animals, and setting up monopolies to control the marketplace are just some of the systemic problems involved in producing 9.8 billion food animals every year in the United States.[41]

Bottom line: a meat-based diet is not sustainable for our planet. Any meat-eater looking to go green should know what Jeremy Rifkin said in his amazing book *Beyond Beef*: "It now takes the equivalent of a gallon of gasoline to produce a pound of grain-fed beef in the United States. To sustain the yearly beef requirements of an average family of four requires the consumption of over 260 gallons of fossil fuel. When that fuel is burned it releases 2.5 tons of additional carbon dioxide into the atmosphere—as much carbon dioxide as the average car emits in six months of normal operation."

Stunning, isn't it? And, by the way, don't forget about all the petroleum-based products (plastic, foam, etc.) used to package your meat. If you really want to stop global warming and leave little to no carbon footprint in your daily life, you have to look at what's on your plate. If you continue to support one of the biggest polluters and destroyers of the planet's ecological systems because you want to ingest dead animals, then you're not part of the solution, you're part of the problem. And if we don't change course soon, we are truly headed up shit creek without a paddle.

WTF IS THAT STENCH?

I was recently on tour with my band in California, driving north on Interstate 5 and about two hours outside Los Angeles when a smell permeated my nostrils that was so bad I wanted to fucking barf on the spot. At first I thought our roadie might have cut the cheese again, but then as we grew closer to the source I knew there was no way even he could produce that level of vile, nauseating, putrid stench. Then we arrived. I saw hundreds of thousands of cows crammed together for miles on end and huge lagoons of their urine and feces. You wanna talk about a hellish planet? Seriously, a month later I still had the taste of that stuck in the back of my throat.

You may have never heard of a CAFO (Concentrated Animal Feeding Operation), but if you've ever driven past one, like me, I bet you've smelled one. A CAFO is like a high-volume assembly line meant to get animals to slaughter quicker and bigger than ever before. What they do is cram as many animals into as small a space as possible, restrict their movement, and pump them full of food (corn, soy, and other grains these animals would not naturally eat) and drugs to try to fight off the infection and disease that would naturally come from that diet and those unsanitary living conditions.

Confining tens of thousands of animals to these over-crowded "death camps" is not only inhumane, it's also highly toxic to you and the environment. Why? Because of that old saying "What goes in, must come out," and in this case it's millions and millions of gallons of raw, untreated sewage, which is stored in large cesspools. When you confine too many animals in one place, they often generate as much waste as entire cities. As Michael W. Fox wrote in the book *Eating with Conscience*, "According to one estimate, if the amount of confined livestock and poultry waste produced in the United States each year were packed in box-cars, they would track around the world fourteen times." That's right, folks: the meat industry creates a train of shit that wraps around the globe fourteen times.

Unlike municipal sewage plants, factory farms aren't required to safely process waste—instead, it gets stored in huge, open cesspools, and eventually spreads into surrounding soil and water. This waste contains toxins, including viruses, infectious bacteria, antibiotics, heavy metals, and oxygen-depleting nutrients that are up to 160 times more toxic than raw municipal sewage.

Heavy metals—which are often present in animal feed in concentrations far higher than necessary for animal health—are of special concern. The health hazards resulting from exposure to heavy metals in water for humans include kidney problems from cadmium; nervous system disorders, kidney problems, and headaches from lead; and both cardiovascular and nervous system problems from arsenic, which is also linked to cancer.

In response to these issues, the U.S. Environmental Protection Agency drafted a new regulation known as the National Pollutant Discharge Elimination System (NPDES) Concentrated Animal Feeding Operation (CAFO) Reporting Rule. Proposed on October 21, 2011, the regulation would require owners and operators of CAFOs to submit detailed location information and farm demographics for virtually every farm engaged in the production of commercial poultry and egg products in the United States.

In their comments, the poultry industry responded that making every CAFO location publicly known would make our food supply vulnarable to terrorists. "Making this kind of information readily available to the public puts the safety of the food chain at an even higher risk for acts of bio-terrorism, not to mention the concern for the safety and privacy of the thousands of family farmers who often live at the same location," said John Starkey, president of the U.S. Poultry & Egg Association. Nice try. Trust me, asshole, al-Qaeda doesn't want your millions of gallons of rotten bird shit.

GET A PEN AND KEEP SCORE

So it's probably clear by now that eating meat fucks up the planet. But I'm not done. I want you to know the specifics on how CAFOs spread their poison. Some of the details that follow may be disturbing to you. Or at least I certainly hope they are. Give this a quick read the next time you hit the drive-through for a burger or pony up to the counter at KFC and get ready to order that twelve-piece bucket.

Beef and Pork: One of the world's largest pig farms is in the United States and holds 500,000 hogs in one Utah facility. Beef steers are a bit different; they spend most of their lives on pasture, raised by ranchers, and then are fattened up for slaughter in feedlots with thousands of other steers.

Hogs are the worst livestock offenders to people. The disgusting odor of hog manure travels for miles—making life miserable for rural residents who are unfortunately downwind of a hog CAFO. Stink is the first problem. As anyone who has taken a high school biology course knows, when we smell something, particles of what we smell are coming into contact with our mucous membranes. So the second problem is that the compounds in those molecules have been linked to all sorts of health problems.

Hogs are usually housed in buildings that contain about 1,100 fellow creatures. There are anywhere from six to ten buildings in one operation. All of those send hog urine and excrement to a "lagoon"—a cesspit. The floors are slatted and the waste goes down onto a concrete through that is flushed with water at regular intervals—each hour or several times a day. A different method is to have the cesspit directly under the confinement building, so that the wastes go right into the pit. No flushing. These pits—whether open-air or under-building—are designed so that they need to be emptied out roughly only twice *a year*.

It is waste handling that gives the operators of CAFOs the most problems. Drains get clogged. Waste pits get full at the wrong time of year—no waste application is allowed on frozen ground. Normally, the CAFO operator doesn't have sufficient land space to dump or spray the wastes on—so a permanent easement is signed with neighbors. The waste application sounds like a good deal: the landowner gets free fertilizer and plenty of it. But most of these contracts don't stipulate any sort of notification to the landowner or any limitation as to amount, and, as noted, the contract creates a permanent easement. Even when the land is sold or owner-ship transferred, that pesky spreading agreement goes along.

Proponents of hog CAFOs will claim that manure is the ideal fertilizer and they are right about that. *But*, similar to most things, moderation is a virtue. A few hundred pounds of hog manure is good; a few million tons is bad. The waste coming from CAFOs is measured in tons: 500 million tons annually, to be exact.[42]

Poultry: With a growing number of consumers switching from red meat to poultry, record numbers of chickens and turkeys are being raised and killed for meat in the United States every year. Nearly ten billion chickens and half a billion turkeys are being hatched annually.

Chickens are given less than half a square foot of space per bird while turkeys are each given less than three square feet. Both chickens and turkeys have the end of their beaks cut off, and turkeys also have their toes clipped. All of these mutilations are performed without anesthesia, and they are done in order to reduce injuries, which result when the birds, stressed by their confined living quarters, are driven to fighting. Most of today's meat chickens have also been genetically altered to grow twice as large as their ancestors in half the time. Pushed beyond their biological limits, hundreds of millions of chickens die every year before reaching slaughter weight at six weeks of age. An industry journal explains that "broilers are now growing so rapidly that the heart and lungs are not developed well enough to support the remainder of the body, resulting in congestive heart failure and tremendous death losses." Chickens raised for their meat also experience crippling leg disorders, as their legs are not capable of supporting their abnormally heavy bodies. Confined in unhealthy factory farms, the birds also succumb to heat prostration, infectious disease, and cancer.

There are two types of chicken CAFOs, but both are equally cruel and inhumane. Broiler houses contain about 22,000 birds. That's not too bad when they're first put in as small chicks (best not to know what happens to the dead ones), but when these birds reach two pounds or so, it gets crowded. That doesn't last too long, though. A broiler chicken is hooked into a small cage, placed in a truck, and carried off to be slaughtered at the tender age of six weeks. Broiler house floors are covered with "litter" (rice hulls, peanut shells, straw, whatever is available) and the birds excrete into that. The litter and chicken shit are cleaned out between flocks and the waste spread onto adjacent fields, several times a year, year after year.

The essence of human cruelty to sentient beings reaches its peak in buildings that house laying hens. Usually there are about 10,000 or so hens in each building, with ten per cage. While some buyers of eggs now stipulate that the cages must be large enough to allow the birds to turn around, it's hard to call that an improvement. The cages are stacked five high in pyramid fashion, so that the excrement from the top cage goes onto a metal "roof" over the cage directly below and so forth. Water from above flushes the waste from all these cages into a central pit, where giant perforated paddles move the solids (including broken eggs) into an outside pit, where this mess is then land-applied as so-called fertilizer.

Dairy: Despite the picturesque images on the sides of milk cartons with a lone cow standing in a green field, the truth behind dairy production is anything but sunny. First of all, you may be wondering: Since female mammals only produce milk when they're pregnant, how do dairy cows produce milk all the time? Ah, exactly—they don't. They are artificially inseminated. Dairy cows are constantly kept pregnant to produce milk. They are fed tons of hormones and antibiotics to fight off disease from their living conditions. A normal cow's life is usually twenty-plus years. At one of these milk factories it's three. The minute their milk-making days are up, they are sent to slaughter.

The cows get milked twice a day by machines that grip and pull their udders, causing pain, swelling, and bleeding. The blood and pus then goes into the milk, but is kept from your sight by pasteurization, and of course more drugs are needed to fight infection in the udders.

A dairy cow excretes about twenty pounds of manure per day. Dairy CAFOs produce millions of tons of raw sewage that are polluting the land and the air with crap like ammonia, hydrogen sulfide, and particulate matter, things known to be serious health risks to our respiratory functions. Actually, according to the EPA the air around these CAFO operations is dirtier than the most polluted cities in the country.

And here's the dirty little secret the organic dairy people don't want you to know: it's been proven that a lot of the so-called organic dairy cows are raised in anything but "organic" conditions. Because dairy cows are auctioned off as commodities from farmer to farmer, many of them are kept in filthy conditions for years before they get the "organic" stamp of approval.

Finally, let's not forget the amount of resources needed to produce milk. The grain, the water, and the billions upon billions of tons of fossil fuels. So when you add in all the pollution and waste of the industry on the environment, all the suffering of the animals, and the fact that humans aren't even made to drink cow's milk in the first place, is it really worth it to keep buying cartons of milk? I will leave it to you to do the math on that one.

Fish: A lot of people who cut back on their intake of animal protein still believe it's fine to eat fish. I want to debunk that idea right now.

As more doctors and diet gurus have gone on TV to talk about the health benefits of eating fish, more people are buying fish than ever before. Well, in case you haven't heard the news, our oceans aren't doing so well, but fish farming operations across the globe have skyrocketed. Aquaculture, or fish farming, has reached epic proportions, growing over 8.9 percent a year since 1950.[43] Maybe you're thinking, "What's so bad about that?" Well, first off, fish farms create toxic nitrogen and phosphorus. Second, the water is treated with antibiotics, pesticides, and other drugs. As for waste from the fish, little is known about how these drugs might affect the offshore marine environment, because the drugs that might be allowed on factory fish farms have not yet been tested in open ocean marine farming situations. But evidence does indicate several serious concerns associated with the use of these drugs.

So maybe you're thinking, "Okay, what if I avoid factory-farmed fish and go for the wild-caught stuff?" Well, sit back and let me tell you a story. Back in 1980 I was in the navy and I would be hundreds of miles out to sea and then along would come these huge garbage barges. They would open the bottom of the barge and all the toxic garbage would empty into the sea. Now, they've been doing that for decades, and still do it even to this day. The ocean is the biggest garbage dump in the world. I mean, where do you think the trillions upon trillions of tons of human garbage from planet earth winds up every day—outer space? Not to mention the latest tragedy: Fukushima and the hundreds of millions of gallons of radioactive water still leaking into the ocean to this day. So don't blame me if you start to glow in the dark after eating your mahi mahi sushi.

Seriously, though, if you want to talk about an industry destroying the largest ecological system on earth—look no further than the fishing industry. Oceanic scientists are ringing the alarm bell and voicing their concern that over-fishing is ruining the planet. That's because the ocean is a very delicate ecosystem; you can't keep pulling out billions and billions of tons of fish from the ocean every day, in some cases wiping out species completely, and think the domino effect will not wreak havoc upon us puny humans as well. We know that all ecosystems are linked; that's just the way it works.

We are not talking about how fishing was done hundreds of years ago in some village in the South Pacific, you know, a boat going out to sea and catching some fish for a small group of people. We are talking about super-killer vessels the size of a football field using sonar and scientific technology to grab every single fucking fish they can get their greedy hands on. As one ocean scientist has put it, they've become experts at hunting and killing fish. These super-killer vessels catch tens of thousands of fish like tuna and store them in fish farms to fatten them up before the slaughter. If you say it sounds just like a feedlot out at sea, well, yes, that's exactly what it is.

I also want to mention that the hands-on mutilation that goes into catching and preparing seafood is pretty fucking sick as well. Boiling lobsters alive, cutting off a shark's fins and throwing it back in the ocean to die a brutal death, cracking oyster and clam shells and sucking them down as they lie dying? Sounds like torture to me. If you did that to a dog, you'd be in jail. I mean every dude reading this probably came out against Michael Vick for his dogfighting, right? If you went on a CAFO tour or spent time on a commercial fishing boat, you would stop eating meat, trust me.

Look, we don't *need* fish or any seafood. When you consider what the industry is doing to the planet, what we are doing to these creatures, and the diseases we put ourselves at risk for by ingesting them, why the fuck would you continue to eat them?

Eggs: Please allow me to shed some light on this industry and what it is you're actually ingesting. As I framed it to a friend recently, "Why would you want to eat the menstrual cycle of a chicken?" His response, "Holy shit, bro, I never looked at it that way." The mental image was enough to make him swear off eggs forever.

Egg-zactly. An egg is just that—an unfertilized egg. And allow me to get seriously gross for a sec (my nickname being "Bloodclot," I feel I have the right to)—it's the equivalent of standing there at your girlfriend's "time of the month" with a bowl, grabbing all that loveliness, mixing it with some red and green peppers, then cooking it and throwing it on a kaiser roll. That's right, my homies and homie-ettes. Sorry if that offends you.

Just like other CAFOs, waste is a huge problem—a henhouse holding one million hens produces 125 tons of wet manure daily. That's just one farm. And the waste of resources is pretty staggering as well: 63 gallons of water are needed to produce one egg, and 23 percent of feed protein is converted to animal protein in eggs.

As for the cruelty of the egg biz, just like in the rest of the poultry business, the chickens are confined in cages and packed together so tightly there's not even an inch to move, and they too have their feet, wings, and beaks clipped. And what happens to the lady chickens once they can no longer produce eggs? Well, let me tell you: they are killed (beaten to death or gassed), ground up, and used for products like canned chicken noodle soup. That shit's not comfort food; it's what's on the menu at the darkest regions of Dante's inferno.

Because the industry primarily needs hens, most of the baby male chicks are immediately discarded after birth, killed alive in giant meat grinders. In Howard Lyman's amazing book *Mad Cowboy*, he describes the "rendering plants," where discarded animals like the male chicks, roadkill, euthanized pets, and sick and dying animals from feedlots are thrown together and ground up. Then the fat solids (which go in soaps, shampoo, and other cleaning products) are separated from the protein solids, which are combined with corn, soy, and wheat and pressed into pellets to create animal feed.

And please don't fall for the lies of the whole free-range and cage-free crap, either. Many of those producers carry out the same cruel practices, and all for what? Because the egg industry tells you eggs are a good source of protein? Listen, do yourself, the chickens, and the environment a huge favor, and make yourself a nice bowl of rice and beans.

BE A SEEKER OF THE TRUTH

I don't know if the information in this appendix has changed your perspective about the food on your plate. I just know that for myself, personally, I want to have the peace of mind that every time I sit down to eat, my meal isn't responsible for destroying the planet's ecosystem or contributing to the torture of some poor creature.

Also, you might want to ask yourself: "Why don't I already know this shit?" Don't we, the public, have a right to know where our food comes from? So you would think, but your freedom of information is in serious fucking jeopardy, as these killing industries have been able to get laws passed in several states that make it a crime to take video footage of their CAFOs. And it is now illegal in thirteen states to publicly criticize corporate food products, under "food disparagement" laws. Because if anyone knew what was really going on, no one would eat what their asses are peddling.

The truth is out there. We just need to seek it out through the quagmire of bullshit being fed to us on a daily basis. Use your Stop and Think Mechanism in every aspect of your daily life, especially when you choose what you will eat. Remember, we do not own Mother Earth, we're merely her custodians. So let's put our collective energy and consciousness together to make a profound change. Let's leave this planet in a better state than we found it. WE HAVE THE POWER.

NOTES

1. American Cancer Society 1996 Advisory Committee on Diet, Nutrition, and Cancer Prevention, "Guidelines on Diet, Nutrition, and Cancer Prevention: Reducing the Risk of Cancer with Healthy Food Choices and Physical Activity," *CA: A Cancer Journal for Clinicians* 46, no. 6 (1996): 325–41, http://onlinelibrary.wiley.com/doi/10.3322/canjclin.46.6.325/pdf, accessed December 8, 2013.

2. Sam Howe Verhovek, "Gain for Winfrey in Suit by Beef Producers in Texas," *New York Times*, February 18, 1998, http://www.nytimes.com/1998/02/18/us/gain-for-winfrey-in-suit-by-beef-producers-in-texas.html, accessed December 8, 2013.

3. Centers for Disease Control and Prevention, "Leading Causes of Death," http://www.cdc.gov/nchs/fastats/lcod.htm, last modified January 11, 2013, accessed December 8, 2013.

4. "Trade, Foreign Policy, Diplomacy and Health: Pharmaceutical Industry," World Health Organization, 2013, http://www.who.int/trade/glossary/story073/en/, accessed December 8, 2013.

5. "Irony Alert: Buy KFC's 800-Calorie Soda to Support Diabetes Research," *The Week*, June 17, 2011, http://theweek.com/article/index/216462/irony-alert-buy-kfcs-800-calorie-soda-to-support-diabetes-research, accessed December 8, 2013.

6. "Health Policies and Data: OECD Health Data 2013," Organisation for Economic Co-operation and Development, 2013, http://www.oecd.org/health/health-systems/oecdhealthdata.htm, accessed December 8, 2013.

7. Andrew Martin, "Consumers Won't Know What They're Missing," *New York Times*, November 11, 2007, http://www.nytimes.com/2007/11/11/

business/11feed.html?_r=0, accessed December 8, 2013.

8. "Issue Brief Series: Pesticides," Healthy Environments for Children Alliance, World Health Organization, http://www.who.int/heca/infomaterials/en/pesticides.pdf, accessed December 8, 2013.

9. Pam Belluck, "Children's Life Expectancy Being Cut Short by Obesity," *New York Times*, March 17, 2005, http://www.nytimes.com/2005/03/17/health/17obese.html, accessed December 8, 2013.

10. "Total Unaudited and Audited Global Pharmaceutical Market by Region," IMS Institute for Healthcare Informatics, May 2012, http://www.imshealth.com/deployedfiles/ims/Global/Content/Corporate/Press%20Room/Top-Line%20Market%20Data%20&%20Trends/2011%20Top-line%20Market%20Data/Regional_Pharma_Market_by_Spending_2011-2016.pdf, accessed December 8, 2013.

11. Andrew Pollack, "After Loss, the Fight to Label Modified Food Continues," *New York Times*, November 7, 2012, http://www.nytimes.com/2012/11/08/business/california-bid-to-label-genetically-modified-crops.html?_r=0, accessed December 16, 2013.

12. "Genetically Modified Foods," American Academy of Environmental Medicine, May 8, 2009, http://www.aaemonline.org/gmopost.html, accessed December 16, 2013.

13. Charles M. Benbrook, "Impacts of Genetically Engineered Crops on Pesticide Use in the U.S.—The First Sixteen Years," *Environmental Sciences Europe* 24, no. 24 (2012), doi:10.1186/2190-4715-24-24, http://www.enveurope.com/content/24/1/24, accessed December 8, 2013.

14. Ellen Crean, "Toxic Secret," CBS News, November 7, 2002, http://www.cbsnews.com/news/toxic-secret-07-11-2002/, accessed December 8, 2013.

15. "Antioxidants and Cancer Prevention," National Cancer Institute, http://www.cancer.gov/cancertopics/factsheet/prevention/antioxidants, last reviewed September 13, 2013, accessed December 8, 2013.

16. "Hazardous Substances and Hazardous Waste: Fact Flash," Environmental Protection Agency, http://www.epa.gov/superfund/students/clas_act/haz-ed/ff_01.htm, last updated August 9, 2011, accessed December 16, 2013.

17. V. Lobo, A. Patil, A. Phatak, and N. Chandra, "Free Radicals, Antioxidants and Functional Foods: Impact on Human Health," *Pharmacognosy Reviews* (July–December 2010): 118–26, http://www.ncbi.nlm.nih.gov/pmc/articles/PMC3249911/, accessed December 8, 2013.

18. "CDC Estimates 1 in 88 Children in United States Has Been Identified as Having an Autism Spectrum Disorder," Centers for Disease Control and Prevention, March 29, 2012, http://www.cdc.gov/media/releases/2012/p0329_autism_disorder.html, accessed December 8, 2013.

19. Vinay Kumar, Abul K. Abbas, Nelson Fausto, and Richard N. Mitchell, *Robbins Basic Pathology*, 8th ed. (Philadelphia: Saunders Elsevier, 2007), pp. 348–51.

20. "One in Three US Children Born in 2000 Will Develop Diabetes," WorldHealth.net, November 10, 2003, http://www.worldhealth.net/news/one_in_three_us_children_born_in_2000_wi/, accessed December 8, 2013.

21. "Preventing Childhood Obesity: Tips for Parents," New York State Department of Health, http://www.health.ny.gov/prevention/nutrition/resources/obparnts.htm, last modified June 2012, accessed December 8, 2013.

22. "Red Meat and Colon Cancer," *Harvard Medical School Family Health Guide*, http://www.health.harvard.edu/fhg/updates/Red-meat-and-colon-cancer.shtml, accessed December 19, 2013.

23. Sabine Rohrmann et al., "Meat Consumption and Mortality," *BMC Medicine*, March 7, 2013, http://www.biomedcentral.com/1741-7015/11/63/abstract, accessed December 12, 2013.

24. T. Huang, B. Yang, J. Zheng, G. Li, M. L. Wahlqvist, and D. Li,

"Cardiovascular Disease Mortality and Cancer Incidence in Vegetarians: A Meta-Analysis and Systematic Review," *Annals of Nutrition and Metabolism* 60 (2012): 233–40, http://www.karger.com/Article/Pdf/337301, accessed December 8, 2013.

25. "Chemicals in Meat Cooked at High Temperatures and Cancer Risk," National Cancer Institute, http://www.cancer.gov/cancertopics/factsheet/Risk/cooked-meats, reviewed October 15, 2010, accessed December 8, 2013.

26. "Nutrition to Reduce Cancer Risk," Stanford School of Medicine, Cancer Institute, http://cancer.stanford.edu/information/nutritionAndCancer/reduceRisk, accessed December 8, 2013.

27. "Cancer Trends Progress Report—2011/2012 Update," National Cancer Institute, http://progressreport.cancer.gov/highlights.asp, last reviewed August 14, 2012, accessed December 8, 2013.

28. "Chlorella," WebMD, 2009, http://www.webmd.com/vitamins-supplements/ingredientmono-907-CHLORELLAaspx?activeIngredientId=907&activeIngredientName=CHLORELLA, accessed December 8, 2013.

29. "Pollution from Giant Livestock Farms Threatens Public Health: Waste Lagoons and Manure Sprayfields—Two Widespread and Environmentally Hazardous Technologies—Are Poorly Regulated," Natural Resources Defense Council, http://www.nrdc.org/water/pollution/nspills.asp, accessed December 8, 2013.

30. "The Controversy Over Added Hormones in Meat and Dairy," NYU Langone Medical Center, http://www.med.nyu.edu/content?ChunkIID=90869, last reviewed November 2012, accessed December 18, 2013.

31. Sydney Lupkin, "FDA: Stop Feeding Livestock Antibiotics for Growth Promotion . . . Please?," ABC News, December 11, 2013, http://abcnews.go.com/Health/fda-stop-feeding-livestock-antibiotics-growth-promotionplease/story?id=21175760, accessed December 18, 2013.

32. "Animal Disposition/Food Safety: Post-mortem Inspection," United States Department of Agriculture, January 27, 2012, http://www.fsis.usda.gov/wps/wcm/connect/6d982860-3c8d-4685-8068-6cffd00ae9ec/PHVt-Post_Mortem_Inspection.pdf?MOD=AJPERES, accessed December 18, 2013.

33. A. J. Cross et al., "A Large Prospective Study of Meat Consumption and Colorectal Cancer Risk: An Investigation of Potential Mechanisms Underlying This Association," *Cancer Research* 70, no. 6 (2010): 2604–14, http://cancerres.aacrjournals.org/content/70/6/2406, accessed December 8, 2013.

34. "Report on Carcinogens, Twelfth Edition (2011)," National Toxicology Program, National Institutes of Health, June 10, 2011, http://ntp.niehs.nih.gov/ntp/roc/twelfth/profiles/Nitrosamines.pdf, accessed December 8, 2013.

35. "Dietary Reference Intakes," Food and Nutrition Board, Institute of Medicine, National Academies.

36. Elaine Magee, "3-Hour Diet or 3 Meals a Day?," MedicineNet.com, http://www.medicinenet.com/script/main/art.asp?articlekey=56254, accessed December 8, 2013.

37. "Erectile Dysfunction," American Urological Association, http://www.auanet.org/education/erectile-dysfunction.cfm, accessed December 8, 2013.

38. "Prevalence of Self-Reported Obesity Among U.S. Adults: BRFSS, 2012," Centers for Disease Control and Prevention, http://www.cdc.gov/obesity/data/adult.html, last updated August 16, 2013, accessed December 15, 2013.

39. James McWilliams, "The Myth of Sustainable Meat," *New York Times*, April 12, 2012, http://www.nytimes.com/2012/04/13/opinion/the-myth-of-sustainable-meat.html?_r=0, accessed December 8, 2013.

40. Felicity Carus, "UN Urges Global Move to Meat and Dairy-Free Diet," *Guardian*, June 2, 2010, http://www.theguardian.com/

environment/2010/jun/02/un-report-meat-free-diet, accessed
December 8, 2013.

41. "Putting Meat on the Table: Industrial Farm Animal Production in
America," Pew Commission on Industrial Farm Animal Production,
http://www.ncifap.org/_images/PCIFAPFin.pdf, accessed
December 8, 2013.

42. John Haines, "U.S. Perspectives on CAFO Waste Issues,"
Environmental Protection Agency, National Risk Management
Research Library, http://www.epa.gov/ncer/publications/workshop/
pdf/workshop_abstracts_cafo82007.pdf, accessed December 8,
2013.

43. J. R. Arthur and Jochen Nierentz, "Overview of Production and
Trade—the Role of Aquaculture Fish Supply"(paper presented at the
Global Trade Conference on Aquaculture, Qingdao, China, May
29–31, 2007). Accessed February 5, 2014, http://books.google.com/
books?hl=en&lr=&id=VYpaObP4gyQC&oi=fnd&pg=PA117&d-
q=aquaculture+growth+since+1950&ots=xqlpAALxrk&sig=_PqX-
7nIrB4GLernvhYjgFrHk5HA#v=onepage&q=aquaculture%20
growth%20since%201950&f=false.

INDEX

Page numbers in *italics* refer to illustrations.

acidic vs. alkaline foods, 18–19, 77–78, 98, 101, 103
addiction, 14–16
AFA (aphanizomenon flos-aquae; blue-green algae), 78, 144–45
Agent Orange, 41
aging, 53
albumin, 95
algae, 103. *See also* AFA; chlorella
Almond Flaxseed Burger, 215–16
Alzheimer's disease, 146
American Academy of Environmental Medicine, 41
amino acids, 78
ammonia, 99, 102–3
anemia, 144
Angelica Kitchen, 234, 241
anger, 19

Anthony, Carmelo, 150, 157
antibiotics, 80, 272
anti-inflammatories, 146
antioxidants, 54, 143–44
apple(s), 142
    Cinnamon Cereal, 192–93
arsenic, 61, 265
arteries and veins, xx, 54, 71, 94, 98, 119, 121, 194, 250
arthritis, 146
artificial color and flavors, 74, 114, 141
artificial sweeteners, 74, 111, 140
aspartame, 140
athletes, 101–4
Atkins diet, 112–13, 121
ATP (adenosine triphosphate), 98
autism, 54
autoimmune diseases, 53

Avocado Salsa, Beefless Soft Tacos with Green Salsa Marinade and, 210–12
Awesome, Cam, *87*

Badgley, Penn, 157
balance, 108, 109, 131
bar codes, 45–46
beans
    Black, with Soba Sensation Sauce, Steamed Veggies, and Quinoa, 234–36
    Rice and, 95, 97
    Roasted Vegetable Medley and, 235–37
    Veggie Chili with Corn Bread, 198–201
    White, with Ricotta Pasta, 204
beef, 266–68
beer, 80
berry
    Compote, with Pancakes or Waffles, 196–98
    Peach Crisp, 245–46
Beyoncé, 23
Beyond Beef (Rifkin), 262
BHA, 141
BHT, 141
bioaccumulation, 43
Bisci, Fred, 36, 67, *85*, 98–99, 171, 249–52
blender, 182
Block, Gladys, xiii
blood and circulation, 18–19, 71, 74, 78–79, 98, 101, 119–20, 143, 189. *See also* pH balance
blueberries, 142
blue-green algae. *See* AFA
Bragg, Paul, 67

Brazier, Brendan, 19–20, *86*, 101–4, 178, 182, 192–93, 215
breakfast, 6, 184–98
Burger, Almond Flaxseed, 215–16
Burrito, Teriyaki Chick-N, with Basmati Rice, 205–8
Bush, Reggie, 150, 157

CAFOs (Concentrated Animal Feeding Operation), 263–71, 277
    beef and pork, 266–68
    dairy, 270–71
    egg, 275
    poultry, 268–70
calcium, 18, 101
Campbell, Chris, 101
cancer, xvi, xiii, 2, 6, 50, 53, 59–68, 146, 265
    breast, 44, 250
    colorectal, xx, 60–61, 80
    prostate, 44, 61
Cancer Diagnosis (Diamond and Cowden), 61
canola oil, 39
carbohydrates, 98, 102–3
carbon footprint, 262
cardiovascular exercise, 163–64
Carmine, 114
Carnita Jackfruit Tacos with Avocado and Pickled Vegetables, 218–21
Carrots, Pickled Jalapeños and, 220–21
Cashew Cream, 214
Casserole, Veggie Chicken and Rice, 229–31
celery, 142
cell damage, 53

cellular respiration, 98
Centers for Disease Control and
    Prevention, 54
Cereal, Toasted Apple Cinnamon
    192–93
Chapati, 240–41
Cheeke, Robert, 101
chia seeds, 143
    Nut-Free Tahini 191–92
"Chicken"
    Citrus, and Veggie Stir Fry,
        221–22
    Veggie and Rice Casserole,
        229–31
"Chicken Nugget Beat Down
    Episode" (video), 32
chickpeas
    Hummus, 241–43
    and Lentil Balls with Tahini
        Sauce, 223–25
children, 54–56, 63–64
Chili, Veggie with Corn Bread,
    198–201
chlordane, 61
chlorella (green algae), 78–79, 95, 144
chlorophyll, 54, 103, 144
cholesterol, 95, 119, 121, 144–45
choline, 145
Cialis, 119
Cinnamon Toasted Apple Cereal,
    192–93
Citrus "Chicken" and Veggie Stir
    Fry, 221–22
cobra, 160
Coconut
    Mint Curry, 226–27
    Rice, 222–23
colon, 71–76, 139
colonics, 76–77, 139

Confessions of an Rx Drug Pusher
    (Olsen), 138n
Conscience Cook, The (Ronnen),
    210–12
constipation, 78
corn, 39
Corn Bread with Veggie Chili,
    198–201
cortisol, 20
Cowden, Dr. W. Lee, 61
Crisp, Berry Peach 245–46
Cro-Mags, 15
cucumbers, 142
Curry, Coconut Mint 226–27

dairy, 55, 67, 111, 270–71
Dal with Rice and Chapati, 238–41
Damon, Matt, 157
Danzig, Mac, 88, 101
DDT, 41, 61
dehydrator, 182
depression, 127–28
detoxification, 74–79, 138–39
diabetes, xii, xvi, 2, 3, 50, 52, 54,
    62, 68, 143
Diamond, Dr. W. John, 61
diarrhea, 78
diet, 107–22. See also food; 30-Day
    Diet and Fitness Program
    changing, 35, 73–77
    diet industry and, 109–13
    raw foods and, 114–117
    sex and, 118–22
    smaller meals and, 117–19
digestion, 72, 97–100
Dirty Dozen, 142, 182
DNA, 53
Drogoszewski, Aaron, xxii, 89, 150,
    156–57, 170, 173

drug industry (Big Pharma), 2–3, 6, 29, 34–35, 55, 137–38
drugs and alcohol, 21, 133

Eating with Conscience (Fox), 264
eggs, 67, 269–70, 274–76
Einstein, Albert, 50, 257
emulsifiers, 40
endorphins, 120
endurance, 100–101, 103
Energizing Green Juice, 186–87
energy, 98, 101–2
Engine 2 Diet (Esselstyn), 204
Environmental Protection Agency (EPA), 265, 271
EPIC5, xv, 101
erectile dysfunction (ED), 119–21
Esselstyn, Rip, *84*, 175, 204
Evolution of a Cro-Magnon, xxi
exercise, xxi–xxii, xxiv, 16. *See also* 30-Day Fitness Principles; 30-Day Power Plan
    before breakfast, 130–31
    beginning, 74, 125–35
    body and, 130–32
    cardiovascular terminology, 163–64
    circuit types, 164
    cobra, 160
    military fitness test, 100
    mind and, 127–29
    protein and, 102–3
    push-ups, 159–60
    reverse lunge to balance, 161-62
    single-leg T's, 161
    squat jump to stabilization, 162
    strength-training terminology, 159–62
    what to eat after, 131, 182
    what to eat before, 182

Facebook, 94
farming. *See also* CAFOs
    animal feed and, 41, 80, 276
    factory, xii, 4, 63, 94, 258–65
    land use by crop, 261
    livestock, 80, 94
fast food, 3, 28, 32, 52, 138, 266
FD&C Yellow, 114
fennel
    Fruits and, 216–17
    Salad with Champagne Vinaigrette, 216–17
fiber, 183
Finding Ultra (Roll), xv
fish, 66, 111, 271–74
    farmed, 272
    wild-caught, 272–74
flaxseed, 143–44
    Almond Burger, 215–16
flexibility, 100
fluoride, 141
food. *See also* diet; acidic vs. alkaline foods; green foods; processed foods; superfoods
    chemicals in, 30–31, 51–52
    converting, into power, 97–104
    deciding which to eat, 36
    Dirty Dozen, 142, 182
    Great Food Bamboozle, 138
    healthy choices and, 6, 109–10
    marketing of, 27–30
    organic foods, 46, 140, 142, 145
    profits and, 34
    sequencing, 99
    shopping for, 30, 33, 45-46, 110
    unhealthy, 4–5

food additives, 32, 33, 39–40, 74
  list of, 140–41
Food and Drug Administration
  (FDA), 34–35, 40, 55, 59, 114
food disparagement laws, 277
food labels, 33, 39, 41–42, 45–46,
  52
Food Revolution, The (Robbins), 261
Foster, Arian, 157
Fox, Michael W., 264
Franklin, Benjamin, 68
free radicals, 52–54
Fukushima, 272

ginseng, 145
global warming, 262
GMOs (genetically modified seeds),
  39–46, 80, 114, 140
goji berries, 143
Goldberg, Burton, 61
Gorran, Jody, 121
gout, 99
Grains, Roasted Vegetable Medley
  for, 235–37
grapes, 142
Green Beans Almondine, 237–38
green foods, 77–79, 103–4
Green Juice, 186–87
  fast, 139
  Green Monster, 190–91
  Joint Fixer 188–89
Green Salad with Vinaigrette, 201
Green Salsa Marinade, Beefless
  Soft Tacos with Avocado and,
  210–12
Griffiths, Josh, 178
Grillo, Frank, 173
growth hormones, 80, 111, 140. *See
  also* rBGH

*Harvard Medical School Family
  Health Guide*, 61
HCAs (heterocyclic amines), 62
health, 3–4, 137–46. *See also* diet;
  exercise; food; 30-Day Diet
  and Fitness Program; 30-Day
  Power Program
  changing lifestyle and, 35, 73–77
  daily choices and, 13–16, 53
  detoxification and, 138–39
  eliminating shit and, 139–41
  kitchen equipment for, 132, 182
  making fitness part of, 125–26
  making transition to, 9–10
  organic foods and, 182
  street smarts and, 137–38
  superfoods and, 141–46
Healthy School Lunch Program,
  224
heart disease, xii, xvi, 2, 14, 54, 62,
  68, 94, 121, 250, 251, 265
heavy metals, 78, 264–65
Hemingway, Ernest, 9
hemp seeds, 103, 145
herbicides, 41
high-fructose corn syrup, 39, 140
Hinds, Jon, 169
Hippocrates Health Institute, 65
Holmes, Keith, 101
hormones, 63
Howard, Desmond, 101
Hugo, Victor, 56
hummus, 241–43
hydrogenated oil, 30, 39–40, 74,
  141
hypertension, xx, 62

immune system, 18, 41, 63, 68, 78,
  99, 143

inflammation, 103
inositol, 145
International Panel of Sustainable
    Resource Management, 260
intestines, 98
intoxication, 16–17
iron, 79
Ironman Stew, 208–10
Ironman triathlons, xxi, 15, 78, 101,
    128–29, 156
irradiation, 139–40

Jackfruit Carnita Tacos with
    Avocado and Pickled
    Vegetables, 218–21
Jalapeños, Pickled Carrots and,
    220–21
Jay-Z, 23
Johns Hopkins Center for a Livable
    Future, 261
Joint Fixer Green Juice, 188–89
joint problems, 77
Joseph, John, *90–91*
juice, 6, 182
    Energizing Green, 186–87
    Green Monster, 190–91
    Joint Fixer Green 188–89
    Nut-Free Tahini Chia, 191–92
    raw, 99
    Skin Trip, 189–90
    wheatgrass, 78–79, 139, 143
juicer, 182
Just Food (McWilliams), 259
Juvenile Diabetes Research
    Foundation, 3

kale, 103, 142
    Chips, 243–45
Kidney problems, 5–6, 101, 265

KISS (Keep It Simple, Stupid),
    131–32
Kordich, Jay, 4–5, 67
Kulvinskas, Viktoras P., 65

LaLanne, Jack, 67
Lanou, Amy, 121
laxatives, 76
lecithin, 39, 40, 95, 145
Lentil and Chickpea Balls with
    Tahini Sauce, 223–25
Lester, Jason, xv
lettuce, 142
Lewis, Carl, 101
lingans, 144
lungs, 98
Lyman, Howard, xiii, 275

maca, 145
macro-psychotics, 24
Mad Cowboy, The (Lyman), xiii,
    275–76
mad cow disease, xiii
magnesium, 144
Mahler, Mike, *86*, 101, 171
maltodextrin, 114
marathon, 104
Marine Corps Marathon, xxi
masculinity, x, xiv
McEachern, Leslie, 234, 241
McWilliams, James, 259
meat
    CAFOs and, 263–71
    cancer and, 60–62
    environment and, 257–62
    grass-fed, 259
    industry, 81, 261–62
    macho myth and, xix-xx, 100
    nitrogen gas and, 99

meat *(continued)*
    organic, free-range, 259–60
    replacing, with plant foods,
      73–74
    school lunches and, 55
    toxins in, 66, 80–81
Men's Fitness, xv
mental toughness, 128. *See also*
    mind; positive mental attitude
    training tips (MTT), 151, 154,
      165–79
Messina, Chris, 157
metabolism, xxiv, 78, 101, 130
milk, 271
Mims, Orion, 166
mind, 127–29. *See also* mental
    toughness; positive mental
    attitude
minerals, 103
Mint Coconut Curry, 226–27
Miracle Cleanse Diet, 108
Mitchener, Erika, 166
Monsanto, 41–46
Moses, Edwin, 101
MSG, 114, 140
MSM (methylsulfonylmethane), 77
muscular stabilization, 153

Narcotics Anonymous, 7
National Cancer Institute, 64
National Pollutant Discharge
    Elimination System (NPDES)
    Concentrated Animal Feeding
    Operation (CAFO) Reporting
    Rule, 265
nectarines, 142
nervous system, 265
nitrates, nitrites, and nitrosamines,
    61, 80–82, 141

nitrogen gas, 99
non-GMO labels, 42
    Shopping Guide, 45–46
Null, Gary, 65
Nut-Free Tahini Chia, 191–92
Nutrisystem, 113
NYC Triathlon, *90*

obesity, xii, xvi, 149–50, 250
olestra, 141
Olsen, Gwen, 138n
omega-3 fatty acids, 143, 145
Oprah, xiii
organic foods, 46, 140, 142, 145
osteoporosis, 101
overfishing, 273

PAHs (polycyclic aromatic
    hydrocarbons), 62
Pancakes with Fresh Mixed Berry
    Compote, 196–98
parasites, 76
Pasta
    Spaghetti with Veggie No-
      Meatballs, 231–34
    White Bean Ricotta, 204
PCBs, 41, 43
peaches, 142
    Berry Crisp, 245–46
Pearl, Bill, 101
Perrine, Mike, 237–38
personal hygiene products, 63
pesticides, 30, 41, 44, 55, 62, 63,
    111, 272
pH balance, 18–19, 78, 101
Physicians Committee for
    Responsible Medicine
    (PCRM), 120
phytonutrients, 132

Pierson, Joy, 224
Pineda, Jorge, 223
plant-based diet
    cancer risk reduced by, 62
    cooking habits for, 183–84
    iron and, 79
    monitoring daily food and, 110
    pH balance and, 18–19
    protein sources, 95–97
    recipes for, 181–246
    switching to, xiv–xvi, xxii–xxiii
    "vegan" word and, 22–25
pork, 266–68
Posilac, 44. See also rBGH
positive mental attitude (PMA), 118,
    129. See also mental toughness;
    mind
potassium bromate, 141
potatoes, 142
    Baked, with Roasted Vegetable
        Medley, 235–37
Potenza, Bart, 224
poultry industry, 265, 268–70
Prabhupada, A. C. Bhaktivedanta
    Swami, 135, 167
preservatives, 30, 74
Pressfield, Steven, 9
prevention, 50–51, 68, 79–81
processed foods, 20, 32, 35, 53, 74,
    141, 183
propyl gallate, 141
prostate cancer, 44, 61
protein, 6
    additives, 40
    athletic performance and,
        100–104
    excess, 101
    myths, xix–xx, 93–104
    sources, 103–4

protein shakes, 100
    Endurance Smoothie, 185–86
protein supplements, 100
psoriasis, 76
push-ups, 159–60

Quillin, Peter, 157
quinoa, 95, 229
    Soba Sensation Sauce with
        Steamed Veggies, Black Beans,
        and, 234–36
    Sweet-and-Sour Tofu Balls over,
        227–29

raw foods, 99, 114–16, 139
rBGH (recombinant bovine growth
    hormone), 30, 41, 44, 140
rebounders, 131
recipes, 181–246
    breakfast, 184–98
    lunch and dinner, 198–241
    snacks and dessert, 241–46
resistance, 8–10
resistance training, 152–53
reverse lunge to balance, 161-62
rice
    Basmati, 207–8, 239
    beans and, 95, 97
    Coconut, 222–23
    Dal and Chapati with, 238–41
    sprouted brown, protein, 144
    Teriyaki Chick-N Burrito with,
        205–8
    Veggie Chicken Casserole with,
        229–31
Ricotta White Bean Pasta, 204
Rifkin, Jeremy, 262
Robbins, John, 261
Rockwell, Sam, 157

Roll, Rich, *88*, 101, 167, 177
Ronnen, Tal, 210, 212
Roosevelt, Eleanor, xxiv
Roundup, 41

Saccharin, 141
Salad
  Green, with Vinaigrette, 201
  Shaved Fennel, with Champagne
    Vinaigrette, 216–17
salt (sodium chloride), 30, 32, 141
Scared Straight, 1–2
Schneider, Paul, 157
school lunches, 54–55, 224
Schopenhauer, Arthur, 35–36
Scott, Dave, 101
seaweed, 103
seitan, 95
Sensa, 114
Serno, Chad, 216
sex, xxiv, 118–22, 145
shakes and smoothies
  protein smoothies, 100
  Protein Endurance, 185–86
  superfood, 95–96
  Super Power, 187–88
Shea, Maureen, 157
Shields, Jake, *84*, 101
single-leg T's, 161
Skin Trip Juice, 189–90
sleep, 19–20, 132
smaller meals, 117–18, 131
SMART goals, 152
Smith, Jeffrey, 45–46
smoking, 120
Soba Sensation Sauce with Steamed
    Veggies, Quinoa, and Black
    Beans, 234–36
South Beach diet, 111

soy, 39. *See also* tempeh; tofu
soy sausage, 194–96
Spaghetti with Veggie No-
    Meatballs, 231–34
spinach, 103, 142
spirit, 133–35
spirulina, 78, 144
Sprinkle diet, 113–14
Spurlock, Morgan, 32
squat jump to stabilization, 162
Starkey, John, 265
steroids, 80
Stew, Ironman, 208–10
Stir Fry, Citrus "Chicken" and
    Veggie, 221–22
St. Jude's Children's Hospital, 55–56
Stokes, Angela, 115–16
Stop and Think Mechanism
    (SATM), 33–34, 110, 138, 277
strawberries, 142
strength, 100
strength training, 159–62
stress, 17–21
sugar, 30, 32, 39, 74, 141
sugar beets, 39
sulfites, 141
superfoods, 141–46
  shake, 95–96
  Super Power Shake, 187–88
Super Size Me (film), 32
Survival into the 21st Century
    (Kulvinskas), 65
Sweet-and-Sour Tofu Balls over
    Quinoa, 227–29

tacos
  Beefless Soft, with Green Salsa
    Marinade and Avocado Salsa,
    210–12

Jackfruit Carnita with Avocado and Pickled Vegetables, 218–21
tahini
  Nut-Free Chia, 191–92
  Sauce, with Chickpea and Lentil Balls, 223–25
talk test, 163–64
tempeh, 95
Teriyaki Chick-N Burrito with Basmati Rice, 205–8
Thacker, Darshana, 226
30-Day Diet and Fitness Program, 149–79
  Recipes, 181–246
30-Day Fitness Principles, 151–55
  Can't Fire Cannon from Canoe, 152–53
  Can't vs. Won't, 153–54
  Smart Goals, 152
  Training Weaknesses vs. Strengths, 153
30-Day Power Plan, 164
  eccentric phase and, 155
  Evaluation Circuit, 157–59
  4/2/1 tempo and, 155
  glossary and how-to, 159–64
  Horizontal Load Circuit, 164
  Vertical Load Circuit, 164
  Week 1, 164–68
  Week 2, 168–71
  Week 3, 172–75
  Week 4, 175–79
  Zones 1,2, and 3, defined, 163–64
Thoreau, Henry David, xi, xvi
Thrive (Brazier), 20, 192–93
thyroid, 143
tocopherol, 40

tofu, 95
  Barbecued, 202–4
  Scramble with Breakfast Sausage, 194–96
  Sweet-and-Sour Balls over Quinoa, 227–29
Tomato Bisque with Cashew Cream, 212–14
toxins (WMDs), 51–56
  avoiding, 53–54
  cancer and, 61–63
  colon and, 72–75
  detoxing and, 74–79, 138–39
  green foods and, 77–79
  kids and, 54–56
trans fats, 141
Triathlete, 14
triathlons, xv, xxi, 15, 21, 78, *90*, 101, 104, 128–29, 156
truth
  seeking, 276–77
  three phases of, 35–36
Tuck, Justin, 150, 157
turmeric, 146

ulcers, 78
Ultraman World Championships, xv
United Nations
  Environment Programme, 260
  World Food Conference, 144
urea and uric acid, 99
U.S. Department of Agriculture (USDA), 41, 55, 80, 96
U.S. Poultry & Egg Association, 265

Vance, Todd, 169, 176
Vedas, 133–34

vegetables
  Almond Flaxseed Veggie Burgers,
    215–16
  burgers, 95
  cooking, 132
  Ironman Stew, 208–10
  Roasted, Medley for Grains,
    Beans, or Baked Potatoes,
    235–37
  Spaghetti with Veggie No-
    Meatballs, 231–34
  Steamed, with Soba Sensation
    Sauce, with Steamed Quinoa,
    and Black Beans, 234–36
  Veggie Chili with Corn Bread,
    198–201
  Veggie Chicken and Rice
    Casserole, 229–31
  Veggie Citrus "Chicken" and Stir
    Fry, 221–22
veggie juices. *See* Green Juice; juice
Vermont, 46

Viagra, 119, 121
  "nature's," 145
Vick, Michael, 274
Vinaigrette, 202
  Mandarin, 217

Waffles with Fresh Mixed Berry
  Compote, 196–98
Ward, "Irish Micky," 157
War of Art, The (Pressfield), 9
water, 99, 139
wheatgrass juice, 78–79, 139, 143
Wilder, Deontay, 157
Wilks, James "Lightning," *87*, 179
wine, 80

yoga, 133, 134
Your Healthy Journey (Bisci), 98

Zone diet, 112
zones, defined, 163–64